Gy Endocrinology and Infertility for the House Officer

BOOKS IN THE HOUSE OFFICER SERIES

Burn Care for the House Officer

Cardiology for the House Officer, Second Edition

Clinical Pathology for the House Officer

Critical Care Medicine for the House Officer

Dermatology for the House Officer, Second Edition

Diabetes Mellitus for the House Officer

Diagnostic Radiology for the House Officer

Emergency Medicine for the House|Officer

Emergency Psychiatry for the House Officer

Endocrinology for the House Officer

Hematology for the House Officer, Second Edition

Infectious Disease for the House Officer

Neurology for the House Officer, Third Edition

Neurosurgical Management for the House Officer

Obstetrics for the House Officer

Pediatric Cardiology for the House Officer

Pediatric Neurology for the House Officer, Second Edition

Psychiatry for the House Officer, Second Edition

Respiratory Medicine for the House Officer, Second Edition

Therapeutic Radiology for the House Officer

Vascular Surgery for the House Officer

BOOKS IN THE CASE STUDIES FOR THE HOUSE OFFICER SERIES

Case Studies in Cardiology for the House Officer

Case Studies in Endocrinology for the House Officer

Case Studies in Neurology for the House Officer

Case Studies in Neurosurgery for the House Officer

Case Studies in Psychiatry for the House Officer

Gynecologic Endocrinology and Infertility for the House Officer

Anne Colston Wentz, M.D.

With Contributions by
Carl M. Herbert III, M.D.
George A. Hill, M.D.
B. Jane Rogers, Ph.D.
and
Kevin G. Osteen, Ph.D.

(C-FARR) Center for Fertility and Reproductive Research
Division of Reproductive Endocrinology
Vanderbilt University Medical Center
Nashville, Tennessee

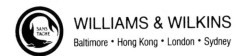

WILLIAMS & WILKINS
Baltimore • Hong Kong • London • Sydney

Editor: Nancy Collins
Associate Editor: Carol Eckhart
Copy Editor: Shelley Potler
Design: JoAnne Janowiak
Production: Raymond E. Reter

Library of Congress Cataloging in Publication Data

Gynecologic endocrinology and infertility for the house officer.
  (The House officer series)
  Includes bibliographies and index.
  1. Endocrine gynecology—Handbooks, manuals, etc. 2. Infertility, Female—Hand-
books, manuals, etc. I. Wentz, Anne Colston, 1940–   . II. Series. [DNLM:
1. Endocrine Diseases—diagnosis—handbooks. 2. Endocrine Diseases—therapy—
handbooks. 3. Genital Diseases, Female—diagnosis—handbooks. 4. Genital Diseases,
Female—therapy—handbooks. 5. Infertility, Female—handbooks. WP 39 G997]
RC159.G97 1987 618.1'78 87-10693
ISBN 0-683-08931-5

88 89 90 91   10 9 8 7 6 5 4 3

Preface

This manual is intended for the guidance of house staff, medical students and Fellows who see patients with reproductive problems. Its purpose is to serve as an outline for evaluation and therapy, and not as a textbook. Tests and procedures are described to ensure a uniform means of data collection. A suggested outline for diagnosis and for interpretation of test results is provided. However, no flow sheet or routine set or orders can be considered absolute for every situation. Although we think that making the correct diagnosis is essential to proper patient management, we know of many alternative routes to arrive at the same solution. We hope this Manual will be useful to arriving at a conclusion, and that it will foster a creative approach to the solution.

Anne Colston Wentz, M.D.
January, 1987

Acknowledgment

The authors thank the many people who have helped with preparation of the manuscript and its illustrations. Drs. Beverly L. Brodie and Liliana R. Kossoy, Fellows in Reproductive Endocrinology, offered useful suggestions. We are grateful to Charlene McDowell, Ruth Robertson, Eilease Preston, and particularly to Beverly Steele who coordinated the effort.

This book is dedicated to Georgeanna Seegar Jones, M.D.

Contents

Contents

Chapter 1

The Ovarian Cycle and Steroidogenesis

George A. Hill, M.D.

INTRODUCTION

The ovarian cycle can be divided into two parts, the follicular phase and the luteal phase. During the follicular phase, the goal is development of a single dominant follicle. The predominant hormone secreted is estradiol (E_2). During the luteal phase, progesterone (P_4) is the predominant hormone secreted. This produces changes in the endometrium to allow implantation of an embryo. Complex interactions between follicle stimulating hormone (FSH), luteinizing hormone (LH), E_2, P_4, and neuropeptides are required for a normal menstrual cycle to ensue.

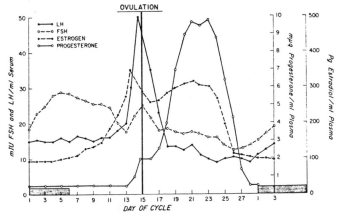

Hormonal changes during the menstrual cycle (Reproduced with permission, American Journal of Obstetrics and Gynecology)

1

2

FOLLICULAR PHASE

Primordial Follicle

1. The primordial follicle consists of an oocyte arrested in the diplotene stage of meiotic prophase, surrounded by a single layer of granulosa cells.

Preantral Follicle

1. Development to the preantral stage is independent of gonadotropins. However, continued growth and development of the follicle beyond the preantral stage requires gonadotropin stimulation.
2. The oocyte has now enlarged and is surrounded by the zona pellucida. During the mid to late luteal phase of the prior menstrual cycle, E_2 decreases. This, in combination with a decrease in the protein "inhibin," leads to an increase in FSH. Granulosa cells proliferate, and the theca layer forms. Proliferation of the granulosa cells is enhanced by E_2 which mediates gonadotropin stimulation of preantral follicle growth. The granulosa cells at all times contain receptors for FSH and thus can respond to the increase in FSH.
3. Early follicular phase and preovulatory phase functions of FSH include:
    a. Inducement of granulosa cell hyperplasia.
    b. Stimulation of FSH receptor synthesis.
    c. Stimulation of LH receptor synthesis.
    d. Stimulation of prolactin receptor synthesis.
    e. Inducement of aromatase enzyme activity.
    f. Stimulation of mucopolysaccharide synthesis and secretion.
    g. Stimulation of cumulus expansion by promoting synthesis of hyaluronic acid.
    h. Stimulation of production of plasminogen activator by granulosa cells.
4. Theca cells contain receptors for LH and are always steroidogenically capable. The interaction of LH with theca cells stimulates androgen secretion. These androgens function as substrate for aromatization to E_2 and are also involved in the process of atresia of follicles which do not ovulate.

Antral Follicle

1. The follicle destined to ovulate protects itself from premature atresia by high E_2 production, which increases its

sensitivity to FSH through promotion of FSH receptor
synthesis and binding, stimulating increased hyperplasia of
granulosa cells, and continuing the synthesis of E_2.
2. E_2 levels are increased in the peripheral circulation by
cycle day 8.
3. Estrogen exerts a positive influence on FSH action within
the maturing follicle. It exerts negative feedback at the
hypothalamic pituitary level, withdrawing gonadotropin
support from the other less developed follicles. Therefore,
the antral follicle with the greatest capacity for E_2
production, the most developed thecal vascularization, and
the highest E_2 to androgen ratio in the follicular
fluid becomes the dominant follicle. Other follicles begin
to undergo atresia.
4. FSH decreases to a nadir in the midfollicular phase.

Preovulatory Follicle

1. During the mid to late follicular phase the dominant
follicle is obvious. It continues to increase in size and
concentrates large amounts of steroid hormones within the
follicular fluid. E_2 output increases and reaches a
peak which is maintained for 24-48 hours.
2. LH output begins to rise with an elevation in the amplitude
of the LH pulse that correlates with increasing E_2
levels. This most likely represents enhanced sensitivity to
gonadotropin-releasing hormone (GnRH) stimulation at the
pituitary level.
3. Granulosa cells are fully matured at this time and contain a
full complement of LH receptors. The presence of LH
receptors ensures that the preovulatory follicle is capable
of response to the LH surge.
4. Under the influence of rising E_2, positive feedback at the
pituitary level results in an increase in LH output. This
increase in LH begins the luteinization of granulosa cells,
resulting in a small increase in progesterone production
which can be first detected in the venous effluent of the
ovary bearing the preovulatory follicle 24-48 hours before
ovulation.
5. This increase in progesterone may work synergistically with
E_2 in the generation of the LH surge and is also
essential for the FSH increase that parallels the LH surge.

4

OVULATION

1. The follicle controls its own ovulation by the mechanism of E_2 and progesterone positive feedback.
2. The midcycle surge of LH initiates a series of events within the preovulatory follicle, leading to ovulation, corpus luteum formation, and reinitiation of meiosis I by the oocyte.
3. The physical act of ovulation involves prostaglandin $F_{2\alpha}$ as well as lysosomal enzymes.
4. E_2 levels have fallen markedly by the time LH peaks. This marks the beginning of a shift to progesterone production.
5. The shift in favor of progesterone begins 12 hours before the onset of the LH surge and increases over the next 12 hours.
6. The termination of the positive feedback of E_2 as well as some negative feedback by increasing progesterone may be involved in the termination of the LH surge. LH may also feedback on itself or through down regulation of receptors for GnRH.

LUTEAL PHASE

1. After ovulation, the granulosa cells increase in size and become vacuolated and accumulate a yellow pigment, lutein.
2. Although the function of the corpus luteum is predetermined by the preceeding follicular events, continued LH secretion is required.
3. Capillaries penetrate the inner layer of the granulosa cells bringing low density lipoprotein (LDL) cholesterol which is the precursor for progesterone, the major product of the corpus luteum. However, E_2 is also produced by the corpus luteum.
4. Peak levels of progesterone and E_2 occur 8-9 days after the LH surge.
5. Progesterone output is released in a pulsatile fashion and correlates with LH pulses.
6. Luteal function is maintained for 14 days unless another stimulus such as trophoblastic human chorionic gonadotropin (hCG) secretion ensues to maintain the function of the corpus luteum. E_2 and prostaglandins may all be involved in the regression of the corpus luteum.
7. The next cycle has already been initiated before menses by the FSH increase which begins in the late luteal phase.

Neuroregulation of the Menstrual Cycle: Neuropeptides are involved
in the regulation of the menstrual cycle, and may be etiologic in
amenorrhea and menstrual irregularities related to stress, anorexia
nervosa, and exercise.

1. Opioids are peptides that have analgesic activity and bind
   to opiate receptor sites. They exert an effect on the
   menstrual cycle by their effect on LH. Their major effect
   is to inhibit GnRH pulse frequency.
   a. Opioids decrease LH output from the pituitary by
      their suppressant effect on GnRH neurons.
   b. Opioid-receptor antagonists (Naloxone) increase LH
      output by increasing GnRH output.
   c. Opioids have no direct effect on the pituitary.
   d. Gonadal steroids partially modulate gonadotropin
      output by their effect on endogenous opiate
      activity. β-Endorphin concentrations in
      hypophyseal-portal blood are increased by E_2 and
      progesterone.
   e. Opioids appear to mediate the inhibitory effects of
      ovarian steroids.
2. Catecholamines exert an effect at the level of the medial
   basal hypothalamus which is richly innervated by
   catecholaminergic terminals.
   a. Dopamine inhibits GnRH output.
   b. Norepinephine has been reported to increase GnRH
      output, although recent evidence suggests that it
      may actually have no effect.
3. α-adrenergic neurons appear to facilitate GnRH-mediated
   gonadotropin release.

STEROIDOGENESIS

The basic ring structure of steroids is shown below.

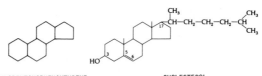

CYCLOPENTANOPHENANTHRENE
RING

CHOLESTEROL

Structures of the cyclopentanophenanthrene ring and
cholesterol.

Cholesterol is the naturally occuring precursor from which all steroids are derived. Cholesterol is synthesized from acetate and transported to the site of steroid synthesis through the bloodstream as low density lipoprotein cholesterol, the preferred substrate for steroid synthesis. Specific high-affinity low density lipoprotein receptors have been shown to be present in the steroid synthesizing cells.

The major groups of steroids are the C-21 steroids (Pregnane), the C-19 steroids (Androstane), and the C-18 steroids (Estratriene). The basic ring structure of the C-21 steroids is shown below.

The basic ring structure of the C-21 steroids

Adrenal Steroidogenesis

The adrenal cortex is composed of three zones, the zona glomerulosa, the zona fasciculata, and the zona reticularis. Their primary products are listed below:

Zona glomerulosa	Mineralocorticoids (aldosterone most important)
Zona fasciculata	Glucocorticoids
Zona reticularis	Androgens

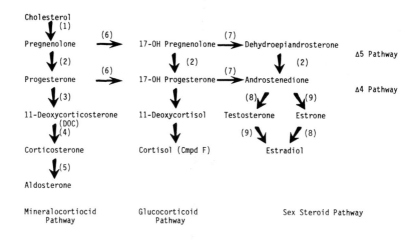

(1) Cholesterol P-450 side chain cleavage enzyme (20, 22 Desmolase)
(2) 3β-ol-Hydroxysteroid Dehydrogenase-Δ ^{4,5}-Isomerase
(3) 21 Hydroxylase
(4) 11β-Hydroxylase
(5) 18 Hydroxylase
(6) 17α Hydroxylase
(7) 17, 20 Desmolase
(8) 17β Ketosteroid reductase
(9) Aromatase

The majority of the cholesterol used for steroidogenesis is derived from the plasma via the interaction of low density lipoprotein (LDL) with membrane receptors of the adrenal cortical cells and subsequent internalization. The reaction

<cholesterol ester hydrolase>
<cholesterol fatty acid   cholesterol   +   free fatty acid>

generally precedes the steps shown in the following figure. These cells also have the capacity for de novo synthesis of cholesterol from acetate. Each of the enzymes is localized within the mitochondria or microsomes (smooth endoplasmic reticulum). Co-factors such as nicotinamide adenine dinucleotide phospate (NADPH), nicotinamide adenine dinucleotide (NADH) and cytochrome P450 are required for these enzymatic reactions. They are not shown, but must be kept in mind when assessing possible enzyme deficiencies in patients.

In the zona glomerulosa, the renin-angiotension system is one of the major controls involved in regulation of aldosterone secretion. Extracellular fluid volume, kidney perfusion pressure, sodium concentration, and the sympathetic nervous system are all involved in the control of renin secretion. Angiotension II is the stimulus to aldosterone secretion in the renin angiotension system. The potassium levels also effect aldosterone secretion directly at the glomerulosa cells.

In the zona fasciculata and reticularis, corticotropin (ACTH) is the trophic hormone for cortisol and adrenal androgen secretion. Cortisol exerts negative feedback control over ACTH secretion. ACTH secretion is also subject to diurnal changes and external stimuli which can be grouped under "stress." Hemorrhage, for instance, is a potent stimulus to ACTH secretion. Adrenal androgens do not have negative feedback on ACTH secretion. ACTH increases cholesterol uptake by the adrenal and also stimulates the conversion of cholesterol esters to cholesterol and cholesterol to pregnenolone. The pathways of adrenal steroidogenesis are shown in the previous figure.

Gonadal Steroidogenesis

Male

Testosterone is the major steroid secreted by the testes. The $\Delta 5$ pathway to DHEA is used primarily. LH stimulates testosterone secretion by the Leydig cells. When testosterone secretion is impaired, LH levels are high. It appears that the major negative feedback control on LH secretion is exerted by a combined effect of E_2 and testosterone.

Female

E_2 is the major steroid secreted by maturing follicles. The granulosa cells are the primary source of E_2 biosynthesis. LH acting on the cells of the theca interna, stimulates the synthesis of androstenedione which diffuses to the granulosa cells, and aromatization to E_2 occurs. E_2 is then released into the follicular fluid and into the peripheral circulation. E_2 is also secreted in substantial amounts by the corpus luteum although progesterone is the major steroid produced by the luteinized granulosa cells. Steroid secretion by the corpus luteum is LH dependent. In humans, the $\Delta 5$ pathway predominates in the follicle for E_2 synthesis but the corpus luteum uses the $\Delta 4$ pathway for progesterone and E_2 synthesis. The pathways to E_2 and testosterone are also shown previously.

STEROID METABOLISM

Nearly all steroids undergo certain types of metabolic changes before excretion into the urine. The metabolic changes include:
1) Ring A reduction
2) Oxidation and/or reduction
3) Conjugation

Ring A reduction. Corticosteroids and androgens generally lose the double bond. The phenolic A ring of estrogens generally is not altered.

CORTISOL   CORTISONE

DHT   ANDROSTANEDIOL

Oxidation-reduction of hydroxyl and oxo (keto) substituents. Most steroids undergo some degree of oxidation-reduction before secretion.

Conjugation. Most steroid metabolites are conjugated to form
glucuronides (glucosiduronates); a lesser proportion form sulfate
conjugates. Steroid metabolism has been shown to occur in liver,
fatty tissue, kidney, and hypothalamus, as well as other tissues.

The metabolic pathways of estrogen primarily involve the two
hydroxyestrone pathway. However, the 16α-hydroxy pathway is also
important. Estriol is the most abundant estrogen in urine and is
the product of metabolism of estrone and estradiol. Most of the
plasma estriol is the result of 16α-hydroxylation of estrone and
estradiol in peripheral tissues. Obesity increases estriol
excretion and decreases the ratio of 16α- to 2-hydroxylation.
Undernutrition decreases the excretion of all metabolites.
Hypothyroidism increases the metabolism of E_2 to estriol while
hyperthyroidism decreases the metabolism of E_2 to estriol. Urinary
estriol excretion does not correlate with plasma estriol levels.
Plasma 2-hydroxyestrone is cleared rapidly from the plasma by red
cell catechol-o-methyltransferase. It is possible that sythesis of
these 2-hydroxy derivatives of estrogen within the central nervous
system modulates some responses of the hypothalamic-pituitary
system.

Metabolic pathways of the estrogens.

Metabolic Pathways of Progesterone and 17-Hydroxyprogesterone

The major route of metabolism of progesterone and dihydroprogesterone is to pregnanediol. The major metabolite of

12

17-hydroxyprogesterone is pregnanetriol. Measurement of urinary pregnanetriol is an important index of adrenal activity in many types of congenital adrenal hyperplasia, but its measurement serves no useful purpose in the examination of disorders of ovarian function unless mild congenital adrenal hyperplasia is suspected.

SUGGESTED READING

Chappel SC, Resko JA, Norman RL, Spies HG: Studies in rhesus monkeys on the site where estrogen inhibits gonadotropins: delivery of 17β-estradiol to the hypothalamus and pituitary gland. J Clin Endocrinol Metabol 52:1, 1981

Ferin M: Neuroendocrine control of ovarian function in the primate. J Reprod Fertil 69:369, 1983

Knobil E: The neuroendocrine control of the menstrual cycle. Rec Prog Hormone Res 36:53, 1980

Lieberman S, Greenfield NJ, Wolfson A: A heuristic proposal for understanding steroidogenic processes. Endocrine Rev 5:128, 1984

Mahesh VB: The dynamic interaction between steroids and gonadotropins in the mammalian ovulatory cycle. Neurosci Biobehav Rev 9:245, 1985

Marshall JC, Kelch RP: Gonadotropin-releasing hormone: role of pulsatile secretion in the regulation of reproduction. N Engl J Med 315:1459, 1986

Quigley ME, Yen SSC: The role of endogenous opiates on LH secretion during the menstrual cycle. J Clin Endocrinol Metabol 51:179, 1980

Short RV: Steroids in the follicular fluid and the corpus luteum of the mare. A "two cell type" theory of ovarian steroid synthesis. J Endocrinol 24:59, 1962

Tsang BK, Armstrong DT, Whitfield TF: Steroid biosynthesis by isolated human ovarian follicular cells in vitro. J Clin Endocrinol Metabol 51:1407, 1980

Wardlaw SL, Wehrenberg WB, Ferin M, Antunes JL, Frantz AG: Effect of sex steroids on β-endorphin in hypophyseal portal blood. J Clin Endocrinol Metabol 55:877, 1982

Chapter 2

Abnormalities of
Sexual Differentiation

Carl M. Herbert III, M.D.

Normal sexual differentiation of a human embryo follows the sequence below:

1. Genetic Sex
2. Gonadal Differentiation
3. Phenotypic Development
4. Gender Identity Acquisition

Genetic Sex

Genetic sex is established after fertilization of a normal ovum by either an X- or Y- bearing sperm. The genetic information for potential sexual differentiation and gametogenesis is carried on the X and Y chromosomes. Two X chromosomes are required for female fertility although one of these is inactivated. A portion of the short arm of the inactivated X chromosome is needed for normal development. The inactivated X chromosome is thought to be the late replicating X chromosome. Retention of an active X chromosome in the male is associated with abnormal spermatogenesis.

The Y chromosome carries structural or regulating loci directing testis formation. A testis-determining gene appears to be located on the telomeric end of the short arm of the Y chromosome. Genes regulating the production of H-Y antigen are located on the euchromatic portion of the long arm of the Y chromosome. H-Y antigen is a plasma membrane antigen originally thought to be the testis determining factor. Although intimately involved in male differentiation, the H-Y antigen is thought to control spermatogenesis, but not total testis differentiation. Genetic material on other chromosomes including the X chromosome may modify or regulate the expression of the testis determining gene perhaps through regulation of a receptor for that gene product.

Primitive zygotes are sexually indistinguishable until after gonadal differentiation. At approximately 6-7 weeks of gestational

14

age, the indifferent gonad arises as an outcropping of the coelomic epithelium. Primordial germ cells which originate in the endoderm of the yolk sac migrate to this genital ridge and are incorporated into the indifferent gonad. The primitive duct systems (mesonephric/Wolffian-male and paramesonephric/mullerian-female) are present in both sexes at this point. Somatic sexual differentiation begins as gonadal differentiation and function occurs. The diagram below shows the time course for male and female differentiation during embryogenesis.

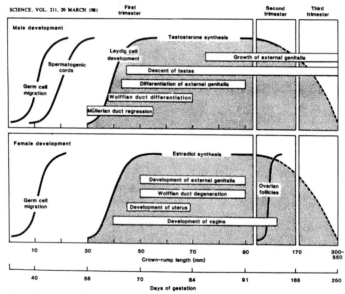

(Reproduced by permission from Wilson, J.D. et al, Science 211:1279, 1981).

Female Differentiation

Under the influence of two X chromosomes or in the absence of Y chromosome material, a primitive gonad will differentiate into an ovary. Germ cells which have undergone mitotic division reach the primitive ovary and are surrounded by a single layer of follicular cells forming primordial follicles. The oocytes within these follicles are arrested in the diplotene stage of prophase of meiosis I. The maximum number of germ cells occurs at approximately 5 months' gestation when there about 7 million present. Atresia reduces this number to 2 million by birth and approximately 300,000-400,000 by menarche. In the absence of two normal X chromosomes, there is rapid atresia with oocyte and follicular degeneration. Differentiation of female external genitalia occurs in the absence of androgens. There are no positive trophic hormones secreted by the fetal ovary which caused differentiation of the female external genitalia. Exposure of a normal female fetus to androgens during differentiation of the external genitalia will cause masculinization.

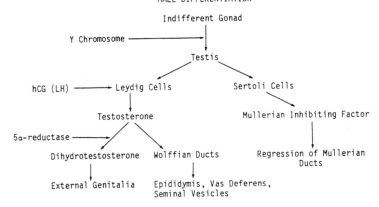

MALE DIFFERENTIATION

Male Differentiation

Under the influence of testis determining factors, the germ cells are enclosed in tubular structures which differentiate into seminiferous tubules and spermatogenic cords. Between these the interstitial cells of Leydig develop which will produce testosterone. Leydig cells have receptors for and are stimulated by hCG (LH). The normal functioning testis produces two important substances for further differentiation of the male embryo, mullerian inhibiting factor (MIF) and testosterone. MIF is secreted by sertoli cells and causes regression of the mullerian ducts. This process is initiated around day 62 is completed by day 77. MIF, however, continues to be secreted until age 2 years and is thought to play a role in testicular descent into the scrotum. MIF functions locally with one-sided ipsilateral effects relative to each testis.

Testosterone is produced by the Leydig cells after day 60. Testosterone production is stimulated by placental hCG which reaches its highest levels during the period of fetal male differentiation. Testosterone acts directly on the Wolffian ducts to cause ipsilateral differentiation of the vas deferens, epididymis, and seminal vesicles. Later during puberty, testosterone also increases muscle mass, growth of the phallus and scrotum, and induces voice changes. Dihydrotestosterone (DHT) is formed by 5α-reductase enzymatic activity on testosterone. DHT is responsible for differentiation of the external genitalia and prostate. At puberty, DHT is responsible for further prostatic growth, changes in facial hair, temporal hair recession, and acne.

There is considerable homology among structures of the male and female genital tracts. The following table lists these structures and their anlagen.

EMBRYONIC DEVELOPMENT OF MALE AND FEMALE STRUCTURES

ANLAGEN	MALE	FEMALE
	GONAD	
PRIMITIVE GERM CELL	SPERMATOGONIA	OOGONIA
PRIMITIVE GONAD	TESTIS SEMINIFEROUS TUBULE SERTOLI CELL LEYDIG CELL	OVARY PRIMORDIAL FOLLICLE GRANULOSA CELL THECA CELL
	INTERNAL DUCTS	
MESONEPHRIC DUCTULES	EFFERENT DUCTULES	EPOOPHORON, PAROOPHORON
WOLFFIAN DUCTS	EPIDIDYMIS, VAS DEFERENS, SEMINAL VESICLES	GARTNER'S DUCT
MULLERIAN DUCTS	APPENDIX OF TESTES	HYDATID CYST (MORGANI) FALLOPIAN TUBES, UTERUS, CERVIX, UPPER VAGINA
GENITAL LIGAMENT	GUBERNACULUM	UTEROOVARIAN LIGAMENT, ROUND LIGAMENT
	EXTERNAL GENITALIA	
GENITAL TUBERCLE	GLANS PENIS	GLANS CLITORIS
UROGENITAL FOLDS	CORPUS SPONGIOSUM, VENTRAL PENIS	LABIA MINORA
LABIOSCROTAL SWELLINGS	SCROTUM	LABIA MAJORA
UROGENITAL SINUS	PROSTATIC UTRICLE PROSTATE BULBOURETHRAL GLANDS (COWPER'S)	LOWER VAGINA PARAURETHRAL GLANDS (SKENE'S) BARTHOLIN'S GLANDS

Abnormal Sexual Differentiation

Abnormalities in sexual differentiation can be classified using genetic, biochemical, as well as anatomical criteria. The following major categories will be used to provide a framework for understanding the diverse etiologies for abnormal sexual differentiation: Abnormal gonadal formation/function, female pseudohermaphroditism, male pseudohermaphroditism.

I. ABNORMAL GONAD FORMATION/FUNCTION

   A. Abnormal Karyotype
      1. Turner's syndrome
      2. Mixed gonadal dysgenesis
      3. Klinefelter syndrome
      4. Polysomy X females
      5. Polysomy Y males
   B. Normal Karyotype
      1. Pure gonadal dysgenesis
      2. Testicular regression
      3. True hermaphroditism
      4. Sex-reversed XX males
      5. Sex-reversed XY females

Abnormal Karyotype

Abnormalities of the sex chromosomes are frequently associated with abnormal sexual differentiation. However, not all karyotypic abnormalities cause development of ambiguous genitalia.

Turner's syndrome describes patients with a 45,X karyotype. Monosomy for the X chromosome results in gonadal dysgenesis which is phenotypically expressed by bilateral fibrous streak ovaries, a lack of secondary sexual characteristic development and primary or secondary amenorrhea. Most 45,X patients are short and frequently have other somatic anomalies.

STIGMATA OF TURNER'S SYNDROME

Short Stature	Horseshoe Kidney
Short Broad Neck	Pigmented Nevi
Low Posterior Hairline	Lymphadema
High-arched Palate	Cubitus Valgus
Epicanthal Folds	Short Metacarpals(IV)
Shield Chest	Premature Ovarian Failure
Coarctation of Aorta	Hashimoto's Thyroiditis
Ventricular Septal Defect	Nail Hypoplasia/Malformation

The genetic material for stature appears to be located on the short arm of the X chromosome while that for ovarian differentiation is located on both the short and the long arm of the X chromosome. A number of structural abnormalities of the X chromosome can lead to development of gonadal dysgenesis/Turner's syndrome including deletion of X_p, deletion of X_q, isochromosome of X_p or X_q, and/or X ring chromosomes. Individuals with 45,X/46,XX mosaicism will be taller, tend to menstruate and be more fertile, and have fewer of the stigmata associated with classic Turner's syndrome. All of these individuals have normal female external genitalia and internal ducts.

Mixed gonadal dysgenesis describes individuals with one streak gonad and one testis which is often dysplastic. The most common karyotype for these individuals is 45,X/46,XY. These individuals may present with a spectrum of phenotypic changes ranging from almost normal female through significant genital ambiguity to almost normal male appearance. The difference in clinical presentation probably reflects differences in distribution of the cell lines. Individuals with female or ambiguous phenotype should have their gonads removed as there is a reported 15-20% chance of developing a neoplasm. The classic neoplasm described is a gonadoblastoma which may contain malignant dysgerminoma cells.

Klinefelter syndrome describes males with one normal Y chromosome and at least two X chromosomes. The incidence of 47,XXY karyotype is approximately 1/1000 liveborn males. These individuals have small testes, azoospermia secondary to seminiferous tubule dysgenesis, decreased testosterone production, elevated serum FSH and LH, and gynecomastia. They are taller than average males and have poorly developed secondary sex characteristics. External genitalia and internal ducts show normal male differentiation. Individuals with 48,XXXY and 49,XXXXY have been reported. They have increased somatic anomalies and mental retardation.

Polysomy X in females most frequently presents as 47,XXX with an incidence of approximately 1/800 liveborn females. These individuals differentiate as normal females and can reproduce normal offspring. Mild mental retardation and occasional physical abnormalities are reported. Individuals with multiple Xs, i.e. 48,XXXX and 49,XXXXX are frequently mentally retarded and have more somatic abnormalities.

Polysomy Y in males most frequently presents as 47,XYY. These individuals have classically been described as displaying sociopathic behavior. Studies have shown an increase in this karyotype among incarcerated males. These individuals differentiate as normal males and frequently are able to reproduce.

Normal Karyotypes

A number of individuals with normal karyotypes will demonstrate abnormal sexual differentiation.

Pure gonadal dysgenesis refers to individuals with either 46,XX or 46,XY karyotype and dysgenetic gonads. 46,XX individuals differentiate as normal females with normal height and no evidence of Turner's stigmata. They lack secondary sexual development and display premature ovarian failure. This can be associated with an inherited form of deafness and is thought to be an autosomal recessive trait. 46,XY (Swyer Syndrome) also presents as a normal female phenotype with poorly developed secondary sex characteristics. The presence of a Y chromosome requires removal of the gonads due to an increased incidence of gonadal neoplasms. This condition appears to be inherited as an X linked recessive or a sex limited autosomal dominant trait.

Testicular regression syndrome describes males with normal 46,XY karyotype who lose their testicles during embryonic or early fetal life. Phenotypic presentation varies between normal male and ambiguous genitalia probably depending on the time frame when testicular tissue is lost. Terms synonymous with this condition include anorchia, agonadia, rudimentary testes, and vanishing testes.

True hermaphrodites have both ovarian and testicular tissues. This may occur in combination as an ovatestes or as a separate ovary and testis. The most common karyotype is 46,XX although 46,XY, 46,XX/46,XY , and other mosaics have been reported. The majority of these individuals are raised as male although there can be ambiguous external genitalia. The testis or ovatestis is most frequently found on the left side and may be either in the scrotum or in the abdomen with the level of descent dependent on the amount of testicular tissue present. Mullerian structures can be present and menstruation can occur. This may present as cyclic hematuria in individuals with male genitalia.

Sex reversed 46,XX males differentiate as normal male phenotypes. Their testes are small and there is evidence of decreased androgen production similar to 47,XXY individuals. Most of these individuals are azoospermic and may carry an autosomal dominant gene abnormality. Current research indicates that a portion of the short arm of the Y chromosome has been transferred to either the X chromosome or an autosome in these individuals. In sex-reversed 46,XY females this same portion of Y chromosome appears to be missing in individuals who are phenotypically female.

II. FEMALE PSEUDOHERMAPHRODITISM

   A. Congenital Adrenal Hyperplasia (CAH)
     1. 21-hydroxylase deficiency
     2. 11β-hydroxylase deficiency
     3. 3β-hydroxysteroid dehydrogenase deficiency
   B. Maternal Drug Ingestion
   C. Maternal Androgen Producing Tumors
   D. Anatomic Abnormalities
     1. Mullerian dysgenesis
     2. Multiple somatic abnormalities syndrome
     3. Single somatic abnormalities

Individuals with a 46,XX karyotype and ambiguous or male genital development are termed female pseudohermaphrodites. With the exception of anatomic abnormalities, these individuals have normal mullerian duct development.

Congenital adrenal hyperplasia (CAH) defines a group of syndromes caused by enzymatic deficiencies in the biosynthesis of adrenal steroids. These enzyme deficiencies result in decreased glucocorticoid production by the adrenal cortex decreased negative feedback, and increased ACTH production by the pituitary. ACTH stimulation of hormone biosynthesis leads to utilization of alternate biosynthetic routes and excessive androgen production. Increased androgen production during development of the embryo causes abnormal external genitalia formation in female offspring. Internal mullerian duct formation and ovarian development are normal. These syndromes are inherited as autosomal recessive traits.

21-hydroxylase deficiency is the most common enzyme defect associated with CAH. There are two forms of this enzyme defect, sodium wasting and no sodium wasting. Sodium wasting individuals produce inadequate amounts of both cortisol and aldosterone while no sodium wasting individuals demonstrate mostly a deficiency in cortisol production. Failure to diagnose this condition in the early newborn period can lead to neonatal death. Diagnosis is made on the basis of significantly increased serum 17α-OH-progesterone or its urinary metabolite, pregnanetriol. Replacement with oral glucocorticoids and sometimes mineralocorticoids will correct this condition. Surgical repair of the ambiguous genitalia is frequently necessary and reproduction is possible.

11β-hydroxylase deficiency is the second most frequent form of CAH. This syndrome is frequently associated with hypertension due to increased production of the sodium retaining steroids

11-deoxycortisol and 11-deoxycorticosterone. Serum levels of these hormones or urinary levels of their tetrahydrometabolites can be used to make the diagnosis. Treatment involves replacement with oral glucocorticoids. Genital ambiguity in female individuals is similar to that seen with 21-hydroxylase deficiency.

3β-hydroxysteroid dyhdrogenase deficiency causes ambiguous genitalia in both male and female individuals. In females, excess production of dehydroepiandosterone causes virilization of the external genitalia. This androgen, however, is much weaker than androstenedione and testosterone, therefore, causing less virilization than the other two forms of CAH. Males affected by this defect have ambiguous genitalia secondary to inadequate testosterone production. Diagnosis is made on the basis of elevated Δ5 steroids including pregnenolone, 17α-hydroxypregnenolone and DHEA. Individuals with this form of CAH have severe sodium loss and should be treated with oral glucocorticoid and mineralocorticoid replacement therapy.

Maternal Drug Ingestion

Certain medications given to pregnant women can cause masculinization of a female fetus. The most common cause of iatrogenic female pseudohermaphroditism is the use of 19-nor progestational agents. These synthetic progestins are found in birth control pills and have been used as progestin supplements to prevent early miscarriage. These progestins are weak androgens so the degree of masculinization is significantly less than that seen in CAH. Progestins implicated include ethistrone, norethindrone, norgestrel, and norethynodrel. Natural forms of progesterone used in oral or suppository form have not been associated with masculinization. Danazol, a 2,3-isoxazol derivative of 17-ethinyl testosterone, is used in the treatment of endometriosis and has been shown to cross the placenta and cause abnormalities in the external genitalia of female infants.

Maternal Androgen Producing Tumors

Androgen producing tumors of the adrenal glands or ovaries in a pregnant mother can produce masculinization of her female fetus. There are a large number of tumors that may produce this (see Chapter 6). Fortunately, the placenta has significant aromatase capability which generally protects a female fetus from these androgenic effects.

Anatomic Abnormalities

Mullerian dysgenesis, otherwise known as Mayer-Rokitansky-Kuster-Hauser syndrome is the absence or abnormal development of mullerian duct derivatives. These individuals have normal ovarian function, normal external genitalia, but no uterus or a fibrous remnant, no fallopian tubes, and a shallow blind pouch vagina with no cervix. These individuals frequently present with primary amenorrhea and go undiagnosed in childhood.

Syndromes of multiple somatic abnormalities associated with ambiguous external genitalia in female children are rare. Reported abnormalities have included abdominal muscle hypoplasia (Prune-belly syndrome) dysplastic cystic kidneys, single umbilical artery, malrotation of the gastrointestinal tract, and various orthopedic anomalies.

Single somatic abnormalities can develop in otherwise normal females. These include agglutination of the labia, imperforate hymen, congenital absence of the vagina, transverse vaginal septum, and various uterine anomalies.

III. MALE PSEUDOHERMAPHRODITISM

   A. Defects in Androgen Synthesis
      1. Adrenal and Testes
         a. 20, 22-desmolase
         b. 3β-hydroxysteroid dehydrogenase
         c. 17α-hydroxylase
      2. Testes
         a. 17, 20-desmolase
         b. 17-ketosteroid reductase
      3. Leydig Cell Agenesis
   B. Defects in End-Organ Response
      1. Androgen Insensitivity Syndrome
         a. Complete testicular feminization
         b. Incomplete testicular feminization
      2. 5α-reductase deficiency
   C. Anatomic Abnormalities
      1. Gynecomastia
      2. Micropenis
      3. Hypospadias
      4. Persistance of Mullerian ducts

Individuals with 46,XY karyotypes and ambiguous or female phenotypes are termed male pseudohermaphrodites. External genitalia and sometimes internal duct development are abnormal.

Defects in Androgen Synthesis

Five different enzyme defects have been described leading to inadequate testosterone production (see Chapter 1). Three of these enzymes are common to the synthesis of adrenal hormones as well as androgens so that deficiency results in CAH as well as ambiguous genitalia. The other two enzymes are only found in androgen biosynthesis. The degree of genital ambiguity may range from mild hypospadias to phenotypic women who masculinize at puberty. Differences in clinical presentation relate to the degree of enzymatic defect and effects of steroids that accumulate proximal to metabolic blocks. All individuals demonstrate mullerian regression and most are infertile secondary to low intratesticular testosterone. These defects are inherited as autosomal recessive traits. Diagnosis is made by measurement of serum or urinary steroids just proximal to the enzymatic defect. Individuals raised as females should have their gonads removed and estrogen replacement given. Individuals raised as males frequently will require testosterone replacement.

Leydig cell agenesis causes a failure of androgen secretion and creation of ambiguous external genitalia. Mullerian structures are not present. Other syndromes which are difficult to separate from Leydig cell agenesis include abnormal LH production and abnormal LH/hCG receptor formation.

Defects in End-Organ Response

Defects in end-organ response are most frequently associated with androgen receptor abnormalities. The androgen insensitivity syndrome or testicular feminization produces normal female external genitalia, no mullerian derivatives, and a blind vaginal pouch. In its complete form, there is little or no pubic or axillary hair and normal pubertal breast development. The testes are normal in size but may be located in the labia, inguinal canals, or intra-abdominally. Testosterone production is normal, however, androgenic effects are not registered somatically. This defect is inherited as either an X linked recessive or a male limited autosomal dominant trait. Receptor studies have shown there are receptor positive individuals with testicular feminization. These individuals are thought to have a postreceptor translational defect. An incomplete form of testicular feminization occurs. These individuals have genital ambiguity with clitoral hypertrophy and labioscrotal fusion. At puberty, they frequently will masculinize with pubic and axillary hair development. These individuals should have their testicles removed before puberty to prevent masulinization and the potential formation of gonadoblastoma/dysgerminoma tumors. During puberty individuals with complete testicular feminization do not masculinize and can undergo good breast development. Therefore, they may retain their gonads through puberty but should have them removed thereafter due to the increased risk for gonadal tumors. Mullerian structures are absent in both forms.

5α-reductase deficiency leads to inadequate production of DHT. This steroid is critically important to the formation of the external genitalia and, therefore, these individuals are born with poorly developed external genitalia. Internal Wolffian ducts are adequately developed and mullerian derivates are absent. At puberty, virilization will occur with increased growth of the penis and development of a masculine body habitus. These individuals do not develop breasts at puberty and have been known to change gender roles from female to male successfully after puberty. This syndrome is inherited in an autosomal recessive fashion and is diagnosed using a skin biopsy from the scotal area. Fibroblasts from this biopsy will show decreased or absent 5α-reductase activity.

Anatomic Abnormalities

A number of anatomical abnormalities can cause confusion about the adequacy of male differentiation. These abnormalities are generally not severe enough to require sex reassignment but sometimes require surgical intervention.

MANAGEMENT OF THE NEWBORN WITH AMBIGUOUS GENITALIA

I. Delivery Room Behavior
   A. Avoid an immediate declaration of sex.
   B. Describe the defect as an incomplete formation, not as sexual ambiguity.
   C. Prevent other announcements of gender (birth certificate, medical records).
   D. Encourage parents to examine baby.

II. History
   A. Take a careful family history looking for:
      1. Family members with similar defects
      2. Unexplained sibling death in neonatal period. (Sodium wasting CAH)
      3. Family members with unexplained infertility, primary amenorrhea or peripubertal surgery.
   B. Carefully review pregnancy history looking for:
      1. Evidence of maternal hyperandrogenism (ovarian/adrenal tumors)

2. Maternal drug ingestion (progestins, oral
contraceptives, Danazol)

III. Physical Exam
   A. Look for extragenital malformations (cardiac, renal,
      gastrointestinal).
   B. Evaluate phallus
      1. Length and width
      2. Erectile tissue
      3. Position of urethral orifice (hypospadias)
   C. Evaluate scrotum/inguinal canals
      1. Degree of labial fusion, scrotal rugation, chordee
      2. Gonads palpable in scrotum or below inguinal ring
         contain testicular tissue
   D. Evaluate Mullerian derivatives/urogenital sinus
      1. Rectal exam to palpate uterus
      2. Ultrasound exam within 24-48 hours of birth (estrogen
         effect on endometrium disappears rapidly)
      3. Installation of a small amount of radiopaque media may
         help define anatomy of the urogenital sinus/mullerian
         ducts.

IV. Laboratory Evaluation
   A. Begin immediately and complete in 72-96 hours.
   B. Cytogenetic studies
      1. Obtain buccal smear to look for Barr body (female) or
         fluorescent Y-body (male)
      2. Buccal smear is helpful but peripheral lymphocyte
         karyotype should be started immediately for definite
         diagnosis.
   C. Hormone studies
      1. Obtain serum electrolytes, 17α-OH-pregnenolone, 17α-OH-
         progesterone, urinary 17-ketosteroids and/or urinary
         pregnanetriol to diagnose possible life-threatening
         sodium wasting forms of CAH.
      2. Measure:

Hormone	Deficient Enzyme
All precursors low	20, 22-desmolase
↑17α-OH-Pregnenolone, ↑androstenediol	3β-hydroxysteroid dehydrogenase
↑Progesterone, ↑DOC	17α-hydroxylase
↑17α-OH-Progesterone	21-hydroxylase
↑DOC, ↑deoxycortisol	11β-hydroxylase
↑17α-OH-Progesterone, ↓androstenedione	17,20-desmolase
↑Testosterone/ ↓dihydrotestosterone	5α-reductase

       3. Diagnosis of other enzyme defects may require
          stimulation with hCG 1,000 units/M^2/day intramuscularly
          for 5 days.
       4. Serum testosterone, E_2, LH, and FSH values may be
    helpful but vary during the newborn period.

V. Gender Assignment
   A. Male gender assignment requires an adequate phallus.
      1. Stretched length > 1.9 cm
      2. Erectile tissue
      3. Lack of severe hypospadias (an ability to urinate while
         standing)
   B. Female gender assigned if:
      1. Inadequate phallus
      2. Functional cervix and uterus present
   C. Complete gender assignment by age 18 months when infant
      gender awareness is established.

VI. Surgical Considerations
   A. Consult experienced surgeon
   B. Phallic/clitoral reduction can be performed early (less than
      2 years of age).
   C. Vaginal construction/repair is better performed around
      puberty.
      1. Increased estrogen (endogenous or exogenous)
      2. Chronic use of dilators is more successful
   D. Remove intra-abdominal gonads/streaks in individuals
      carrying a Y chromosome before puberty.
      1. Individuals with complete testicular feminization may
         have gonads removed after puberty.

SUGGESTED READING

Jones HW, Scott WW: Hermaphroditism, Genital Anomalies, and Related Endocrine Disorders, Second Edition, Baltimore, Williams & Wilkins, 1971.

Josso N: Intersex Child. First Edition, S. Karger AC Basel, 1981.

Simpson JL, Golbus MS, Martin AO, Sarto GE: Genetics in Obstetrics and Gynecology. New York, Grune & Stratton, 1982.

Simpson JL: Disorders of Sexual Differentiation: Etiology and Clinical Delineation. New York, Academic Press, 1976.

Simpson JL: Abnormal sexual differentiation in humans. Annu Rev Genet 16:193, 1982.

Wachtel SS: Errors of sexual determination. Proceedings of the Kroc Foundation Conference. Hum Genet 58(1):1, 1981.

Wachtel SS, Chervanak FA, Brunner M, Lehn-Jensen H: Notes on the biology of H-Y antigen. J Pediatr Endocrinol 1:1, 1985.

Wilson JD, Griffin JE, George FW, Leshin M: The role of gonadal steroids in sexual differentiation. Rec Prog Hormone Res 37:1, 1981.

Chapter 3

Primary and Secondary Amenorrhea

Anne Colston Wentz, M.D.

DEFINITIONS

Amenorrhea is the complete absence of menstruation in a woman in the reproductive span of life. Amenorrhea is not a diagnosis, but rather a symptom with many possible causes. Amenorrhea is termed "primary" in the patient who has never menstruated, and "secondary" in the patient whose menses, after their initial appearance, have ceased at any time during the reproductive span for over six months. Absence of menstruation is to be regarded as physiological prior to puberty, during pregnancy and lactation, after the menopause, and expected during administration of certain drugs (Depo-Provera, danazol, tranquilizers).

PRIMARY AMENORRHEA

Primary amenorrhea is defined as absence of menarche by age 16. However, since menarche is the culmination of pubertal development, evidence of development of secondary sexual characteristics which include breast and pubic hair growth, an estrogenic vaginal smear, and accelerated linear skeletal growth, suggest that pubertal development is progressive and make the tentative diagnosis of delayed menarche more appropriate at age sixteen years. However, it is not always possible to differentiate those women who will proceed to menarche.

Lack of menstruation by 16 years of age warrants evaluation. Growth at adolescence is more a function of physiologic than of the chronologic age and wide variations in patterns occur. A child should be seen whenever her anxieties or those of her parent are brought to the physician's attention. A careful history and physical examination are necessary before one can assess whether further investigation is warranted.

Some knowledge of the normal timing of events at adolescence is needed. The development of the breast bud, called thelarche, is the first sign of puberty, usually occurring at 9-11 years of age. The presence of pituitary gonadotropins and the release of endogenous estrogen by the ovary are implied. Estrogen effects are manifest in the vagina: superficial cells appear in increasing numbers, and the vaginal pH changes to the adult pH of 4 to 5. Shortly after thelarche, appearance of pubic hair signifies the production of androgenic steroids by the adrenal cortex, and this stage is called adrenarche. Axillary hair does not usually appear until the growth of pubic hair is complete. The growth spurt next occurs. This culminates in the onset of the first menstrual period or menarche. In American girls, menarche occurs normally between 10 and 14 years, with a mean of approximately 13 years, at a physiological bone age of 12 or 13 years. Ordinarily, the process of pubertal development, from thelarche through menarche, takes less than 2 years.

Evaluation of the child is then indicated if:
(1) menarche has not occurred by age 16,
(2) secondary sexual development has not occurred by age 14,
(3) height and/or weight are significantly retarded,
(4) 3 years have elapsed from thelarche without menses,
(5) the child or her parents are overly worried.

ETIOLOGIC CLASSIFICATION OF PRIMARY AMENORRHEA

I.   Lesions of Central Origin
     A.   Neurogenic
          1.   Destructive Lesions, Tumors
          2.   Hypothalamic Dysfunction
               a.   Weight-associated
                         anorexia nervosa
                         simple weight loss
                         post-pill low body weight
               b.   Exercise-associated
               c.   Stress-induced
               d.   Psychogenic
                         anorexia nervosa
                         acute emotional disturbances
               e.   Feedback dysfunction
                         polycystic ovarian disease
                         adrenal androgenization
                         obesity
          3.   Hypothalamic Defects
               a.   GnRH deficiency (?)
               b.   Hypothalamic hypogonadism with anosmia
                    (Kallmanns syndrome)
     B.   Pituitary Disturbances
          1.   Destructive Lesions
          2.   Tumors

                a. functioning
                b. non-functioning
           3. Congenital Defects
                a. empty sella
                b. partial isolated gonadotropin deficiency

II. Intermediate Factors
    A. Nutritional
        1. Obesity
        2. Starvation, malnutrition
    B. Chronic Illness
        1. Childhood leukemia, other blood dyscrasias
    C. Endocrinologic Disorders
        1. Thyroid Hypo- and Hyperfunction
        2. Adrenal Hypo- and Hyperfunction
        3. Diabetes
    D. Metabolic Disease
        1. Renal
        2. Hepatic

III. Gonadal Factors
    A. Congenital Defects
        1. Intersexuality
        2. Mosaicism
    B. Premature Menopause
    C. Destructive Lesions
    D. Insensitive Ovary Syndrome
    E. Tumors
        1. functioning
        2. non-functioning

IV. Uterine and Outflow Tract Abnormalities
    A. Uterine
        1. Congenital defects
            a. Uterine absence
            b. Uterine malformation
        2. Infectious diseases
            a. Endometrial sclerosis (tuberculosis)
        3. Traumatic lesions
            a. Cervical stenosis
    B. Vaginal
        1. Congenital defects
            a. Imperforate hymen
            b. Transverse vaginal septum
            c. Congenital absence
            d. Congenital malformation
        2. Traumatic or infectious stenosis

V. Physiologic Causes
    A. Ovarian Failure (Menopause)
    B. Pregnancy (postpartum, lactation)

EVALUATION

The patient's developmental history dating back to pregnancy, labor and delivery must be documented. Evidence of physical or psychologic dysfunction is important. A social and behavioral history are needed to ascertain the child's performance in school and other peer activities. A nutritional history may identify the early anorectic or bulimic patient. Family history of anosmia, or of other affected individuals, may suggest single-gene or other chromosomal anomalies. Height, weight, "wing span," and blood pressure may be useful; body proportions may suggest developmental disease. Skin pigmentation, "cafe-au-lait" spots, evidence of hyperandrogenism and galactorrhea should be detected.

The physical examination should detect neurologic defects suggesting intracranial pathology, and evidence of nutritional or metabolic disease. Determination of secondary sexual development divides patients with primary amenorrhea into those with hypothalamic-pituitary-ovarian maturation with absence of menstruation and those without central maturation.

The pelvic examination should reveal lack of ambiguity of the external genitalia and the presence of vagina and cervix. The bimanual evaluation should demonstrate both the presence of a uterus and the absence of adnexal pathology. It is insufficient merely to document the presence of a vaginal opening, as structural anomalies may occur higher. It is difficult to distinguish between a transverse vaginal septum, a normal but virginal hymen, the short vagina in testicular feminization, and the complete absence of Mullerian development as seen in the Rokitansky syndrome.

LABORATORY WORK-UP

> Obtain at the initial visit (use selectively):
>> height, span, weight, blood pressure;
>> PAP smear plus maturation index;
>> urinalysis with microscopic exam;
>> blood FSH/LH, prolactin;
>> bone age (left wrist and hand film);
>> karyotype;
>> pregnancy test if appropriate.

> Consider obtaining (use even more selectively):
>> pelvic ultrasound;
>> evaluation of anterior pituitary function:
>>> FSH/LH after GnRH stimulation,
>>> TSH after TRH stimulation,
>>> hGH after GHRH stimulation,

ACTH after CRF stimulation,
CT of sella turcica;
thyroid function tests (free T_4, T_3);
17-KS, 17-OHCS, urinary free corticoids;
testosterone, dehydroepiandrosterone sulfate (DS) if
    virilized;
17α-hydroxyprogesterone (baseline and after Cortrosyn);
glucose tolerance test (FBS and 2 hour PC).

Chromosomal diagnosis is highly important in the evaluation of primary amenorrhea with failure of secondary sexual development; if the patient is developed normally, Mullerian agenesis or an outflow tract problem is more likely and the karyotype is less useful. Newer banding and fluorescent techniques are able to identify subtle defects. Therefore, a karyotype should be obtained in the evaluation of most cases of primary amenorrhea.

Evaluation of pituitary gonadotropin output is next. In patients with secondary sexual development, pituitary and ovarian function have clearly begun, and the question to be answered is why it was interrupted, or why menstruation has not occurred. Patients with failure of secondary sexual development have not had the onset of ovarian function and the question is whether the cause is ovarian or central. These patients are ultimately divided into two therapeutic groups, one with no expectation of reproductive function, and a second with potentially functioning ovaries. Very elevated baseline FSH suggests primary ovarian failure. When baseline FSH/LH is low, the response to GnRH can be measured; failure to increase FSH and LH may only indicate that endogenous GnRH output has not yet begun but a positive test rules out a pituitary synthetic defect.

High Gonadotropins: In general, patients with high gonadotropin output have ovarian failure and no expectation of reproductive function. They are treated with exogenous estrogens to induce the development of secondary sexual characteristics, and later regular menses.

The Savage syndrome, with primary amenorrhea, normal secondary sexual characteristics, elevated FSH/LH and oocytes present in the ovarian biopsy, represents a form of ovarian insensitivity that may be responsive to massive amounts of exogenous gonadotropins. Lack of an FSH receptor may be the cause.

Congenital 17α-hydroxylase deficiency also has elevated gonadotropins as this enzyme deficiency prevents sex steroid synthesis. The patient has no secondary sexual development, normal female external genitalia (if 46XX and ambiguous external genitalia if 46XY), hypertension, enlarged ovaries, and high circulating levels of progesterone. This entity is best treated with suppressive doses of adrenal corticosteroids. Fertility is theoretically possible.

Normal or Low Gonadotropins. Diagnostic studies indicate that most patients in this category have a hypothalamic, not pituitary, defect. Tests designed to differentiate between these etiologies usually cannot differentiate delayed puberty from hypothalamic hypogonadism.

GnRH stimulation indicates competence of pituitary production and release of gonadotropins. The early pubertal female shows first a response of FSH to GnRH stimulation, later an LH response exceeding the FSH. Patterns similar to those in the normal adult do not necessarily indicate imminent menarche. From a clinical standpoint, provocative testing is usually not indicated in these patients.

TREATMENT

Therapy as always depends upon the etiologic diagnosis. If the reason for failure to develop secondary sexual characteristics is identified, and its treatment undertaken, pubertal development usually follows rapidly. Examples include patients with thyroid dysfunction and congenital adrenal hyperplasia, although premature epiphyseal fusion may prevent a normal growth spurt in CAH patients. In patients in whom the prognosis for spontaneous development and menstruation is negligible, a regimen of estrogen can be begun to develop secondary sexual characteristics.

Rapid Method: Premarin, 1.25-2.5 mg given cyclically days 1-25 until menstruation begins; add Provera, 10 mg, days 11-25.

Slow Method: Ethinyl estradiol, 10-20 mg, or Premarin, 0.3 mg continuously for 3 months, double the dose for 3 months, and then begin cyclic estrogen days 1-25, and add progestin on days 16-25 after at least 6 months, primarily to induce menstruation, but also to protect the endometrium from a continuous estrogen stimulation.

SECONDARY AMENORRHEA

Secondary amenorrhea is defined as the absence of menses for greater than 6 months in a woman who has previously had menstrual periods. It is to be differentiated from oligomenorrhea, in which the patient has irregular periods, most commonly occurring every 2-5 months.

The diagnosis of chronic anovulation, which results in secondary amenorrhea, implies that primary ovarian failure has not occurred (although determining this is a first priority in diagnosis), and that the system can be reactivated with proper management.

Since the history frequently reveals the etiologic cause of the amenorrhea, the following simple classification is useful to follow in the initial diagnostic approach. There is considerable overlap between categories.

ETIOLOGIC CLASSIFICATION

The classification is identical to that for primary amenorrhea, except for those entities (uterine absence) that would have presented as failure of the onset of menstruation.

EVALUATION OF SECONDARY AMENORRHEA

The history is the most important examination in the evaluation of secondary amenorrhea. "Set the setting" of the amenorrhea, not at the time of the first missed menses, but rather in the weeks or months preceding it. Evaluate for pregnancy exposure, malnutrition, emotional trauma, and hot flashes. Specifically question the patient for symptomatology of intermediate or central disease. The etiology will be revealed by the history 80% of the time, but the right questions have to be asked.

The physical and pelvic examinations serve to confirm the history. Necessary laboratory evaluation is therefore substantially decreased, and well chosen tests serve to document the diagnosis.

Particular clues to the etiology revealed on physical examination include: body habitus, evidence of weight gain or loss, skin pigmentation (tanning, carotenemia), hair loss or hirsutism, striae or bruising, neurologic reflexes, galactorrhea, and so forth.

Clues observed on pelvic examination determine whether ovarian hormone output is or is not active. Carefully evaluate cervical mucus and the vaginal mucosa to assess the estrogen milieu. If a patient has abundant estrogenic cervical mucus, her ovaries are putting out estrogen, her pituitary is putting out FSH and LH to stimulate the ovary, and the hypothalamus must be competent to release GnRH to stimulate the pituitary. This patient is not cycling. She has a continuous estrogen stimulation to her endometrium and can develop endometrial hyperplasia and/or dysfunctional uterine bleedling (DUB). Typically she has an elevated LH, low or normal FSH, increased testosterone and androstenedione, and fits the pattern for polycystic ovarian disease (PCOD).

Most patients diagnosed to have an autonomous estrogen-recruiting ovarian tumor present with irregular bleeding and spotting, not amenorrhea. Diagnostic clues include: unilateral adnexal mass, profuse amounts of cervical mucus, very suppressed serum FSH levels and normal or slightly low LH levels. Estrogen levels may not be massively elevated.

On the other hand, if a patient has an atrophic vaginal mucosa, and no cervical mucus, she is not putting out estrogen. She could have failure at the level of the ovary, pituitary or hypothalamus. Ovarian failure is typified by elevated gonadotropin levels, but lesions affecting the pituitary or hypothalamus are more difficult to differentiate.

Initial Laboratory Studies

1. Evaluate the estrogen milieu: is the patient estrogenized?
2. Draw serum gonadotropins, FSH and LH.
3. Further tests depend on category of patient.

ESTROGENIZED PATIENT	HYPOESTROGENIZED PATIENT
	(Rarely Atrophic)
"Turned On"	"Turned Off"
Lush cervical mucus	Scant cervical mucus
LH/FSH (usually 3:1)	LH/FSH (♦♦or ♦♦)
Testosterone	Prolactin
Dehydroepiandrosterone	? TSH
sulfate (DS)	
Prolactin	
	Sella Turcica Evaluation
Endometrial Biopsy	(coned-down view vs CT scan)
	(CT scan if prolactin ♦)

The three most important diagnoses to be ruled out immediately in any patient with secondary amenorrhea are:

(1) Pregnancy
(2) Pituitary tumor
(3) Premature menopause

A pregnancy test, serum prolactin level and serum gonadotropins are essential initial screening tests. Since unopposed estrogen stimulation may result in the development of endometrial adenocarcinoma, the patient with secondary amenorrhea must be carefully evaluated with this pathologic diagnosis in mind. An immediate endometrial biopsy is not indicated until the above diagnoses are ruled out and evidence of hyperestrogenism is obtained. A serum prolactin (PRL) level may reveal evidence of a prolactin-producing pituitary tumor before abnormalities of the sella can be appreciated; if PRL is mildly elevated, a coned-down view of the sella is usually not useful and a CT scan may be indicated. Patients with other intra- and suprasellar tumors may present with only slightly elevated prolactin levels; we would have failed to diagnose two of our last three craniopharyngiomas if we had relied on coned-down views and not requested a CT scan.

It must be remembered that secondary amenorrhea is a symptom or sign of pathology which must be diagnosed before instituting therapy. In other words, menstruation is only necessary if fertility is desired, and hormonal induction of bleeding is rarely indicated. On the other hand, the hyperestrogenic patient is at risk for the development of endometrial hyperplasia; in this patient, a progestational agent may be used for its antimitotic effects, not simply to induce bleeding.

E. Differential Diagnosis

The differential diagnosis of secondary amenorrhea begins by dividing patients into groups according to gonadotropin levels.

1. High Gonadotropins: These patients invariably have physiologic or premature menopause, secondary to ovarian failure. Rarely, a periovulatory sample may be obtained showing high LH/FSH levels, so ascertain if bleeding occurred within 3 weeks after the sample was drawn and that pregnancy has not occurred. Elevated gonadotropins must be confirmed by at least two additional FSH levels at monthly intervals.

2. Low Gonadotropins: Pituitary or hypothalamic dysfunction is diagnosed. Examples would include panhypopituitarism, Sheehan's syndrome, post-pill amenorrhea, amenorrhea-galactorrhea syndromes, anorexia nervosa, or tumor. Ascertain that bleeding did not occur within 10 days of the sample, as very low FSH/LH levels are normally measured in the midluteal phase.

3. Normal Gonadotropins: These patients will usually have hypothalamic dysfunction with secondary failure of ovulation. Estrogen output may be normal or elevated although noncyclic. Patients who manifest high estrogen output (by maturation index, evaluation of cervical mucus) are likely candidates for the development of endometrial hyperplasia, and should have an endometrial biopsy. If the biopsy shows proliferative endometrium, it is not usually necessary to induce withdrawal bleeding.

4. <u>Variable Gonadotropin Patterns</u>:

PATTERN	DIAGNOSTIC CONSIDERATION
Very high LH, very low FSH	Pregnancy Trophoblastic disease
High LH, normal or low FSH	PCO syndrome
Normal LH, very low FSH	Exogenous or endogenous estrogen
Normal LH, very high FSH	Impending ovarian failure

Estimation of the estrogenic status of the patients will help in assessing the prognosis of spontaneous resumption of ovulation or the success of ovulation induction. A copious, clear, acellular, thin and runny cervical mucus, and cornified cells on the maturation index (0/80/20 or better), or proliferative (not atrophic) endometrium on biopsy are evidence of estrogen production, and by inference, gonadotropin output. Pregnancy is unlikely in the presence of a highly estrogenized cervical mucus.

In the presence of the above, the patient will bleed when given progesterone. This test furnishes some information about estrogenization, but fails to provide important anatomical evidence of endometritis, endometrial hyperplasia, or anaplasia. Its use is neither recommended or indicated but progesterone withdrawal is described because it is used so frequently.

The <u>progesterone test</u> involves administration of progesterone in oil, 50 or 100 mg intramuscularly. Menstrual-like bleeding 4-9 days after administration indicates that:

The patient has a functional estrogen-primed endometrium
Pituitary gonadotropins are adequate to stimulate the ovary to
    produce estrogen
Amenorrhea is probably secondary to failure of ovulation
The patient is not pregnant.

However, simple observation of an estrogenized cervical mucus makes those determinations without the administration of the drug. An endometrial biopsy is needed to rule out hyperplasia.

Menstrual-like bleeding 14 days after injection usually indicates that ovulation was triggered by progesterone.

Patients who fail to bleed after progesterone alone could be pregnant, and must be proven nonpregnant before further testing. With a suspicious history, for example, incomplete abortion with D&C or any evidence of infection following a pregnancy, an estrogen-progesterone provocative test using Premarin 1.25-2.5 mg daily for 10-14 days followed by Provera 10 mg for 5-7 days or a progesterone injection may be indicated. Failure of bleeding or an unexpectedly scant period after estrogen-progesterone therapy and the absence of pregnancy or cervical stenosis diagnoses Asherman's syndrome, intrauterine adhesions or endometrial sclerosis.

"Turned-On" Estrogenized Chronic Anovulation Syndrome

1. Ovarian
   A. Definition of polycystic ovarian syndrome (PCOS)
      1) A heterogenous disorder, a syndrome.
      2) Anovulation, infertility, hirsutism, obesity, and bilateral polycystic ovaries are associated with a number of endocrine disorders including: hyperthecosis, androgen-secreting tumors, Cushing's syndrome, hypothyroidism, chronic anovulation with hyperprolactinemia, congenital adrenal hyperplasia, certain CNS tumors.
   B. Pathophysiology
      1) Etiology is unknown in the majority of cases.
      2) Proposed etiologies include: central dopaminergic dysfunction;
         primary adrenal enzymatic disorder, in partial 3β-ol dehydrogenase deficiency which could become manifest at the time of adrenarche, or an excess of some adrenal stimulating factor other than ACTH (CASH, AASH), causing exaggerated adrenarche; ovarian etiology with hyperandrogenism;
      3) Other associations, with hyperlipidemia, insulin-resistant diabetes, acanthosis nigricans, hypertension plus ovarian hyperthecosis are seen.
   C. Clinical characteristics

Infertility	74%	Dysmenorrhea	23%
Hirsutism	69%	Corpus luteum at	
Amenorrhea	51%	surgery	22%
Obesity	41%	Virilization	21%
Dysfunctional		Biphasic BTC	15%
bleeding	29%	Normal menses	12%

      1) Mean age at menarche, 12.3 years, not different from normal.

    2) Development of hirsutism at or shortly after menarche.
    3) Menstrual irregularity at or shortly after menarche.
    4) Ordinarily overweight.
    5) Positive family history.
    6) Ovaries may or may not be enlarged.

  D. Other ovarian hyperandrogenic syndromes
    1) Ovarian hyperthecosis $\pm$ acanthosis nigricans
    2) Androgen-producing ovarian tumors
    3) Hyperprolactinemia with PCOD-like syndrome
    4) Hypersecretion of LH and prolactin in PCOD-like syndrome

2. Adrenal
  A. Cushing's syndrome
  B. Hyperplasia of the reticularis
  C. Adrenal tumor
  D. Congenital adrenal hyperplasia
      21-hydroxylase deficiency
      11β-hydroxylase deficiency
      3β-ol dehydrogenase deficiency

3. Other
  A. Obesity
    1) suppressed sex hormone binding globulin levels
    2) increased biologically active androgens
    3) increased peripheral conversion to estrogen
  B. Hyper- and hypothyroidism
    1) Elevated plasma thyroid hormone concentration is
       associated with:
       a) marked increase in plasma sex hormone binding
          globulin
       b) an increase in 21-hydroxylase activity
       c) increased catecholestrogen formation
       d) amenorrhea more common
    2) Hypothyroidism is associated with:
       a) increased MCR for testosterone which is due to
       b) reduced sex hormone binding globulin
       c) increased androstenedione to testosterone conversion
       d) abnormal bleeding more common than amenorrhea

4. Management of "turned-on" (estrogenized) chronic anovulation
  syndromes
  A. Depends entirely on the chief complaint of the patient
    1) Fertility
    2) Establishment of menstrual regulation
    3) Treatment of hirsutism
  B. Choices are:
    1) Ovulation induction

      2) Do nothing
      3) Cyclic progestational agent
      4) Suppressive birth control pills
      5) ? adrenal suppression

C. Fertility
      1) Clomiphene citrate for ovulation induction is the treatment of choice
      2) Other modalities include clomiphene plus dexamethasone, and clomiphene plus hCG; bilateral wedge resection is reserved for the patient who has failed to ovulate on clomiphene and human menopausal gonadotropin, GnRH and combinations.

D. Menstrual regulation and hirsutism
      1) Do nothing, which will not treat the hirsutism or regulate the menstrual cycles and could lead to bouts with dysfunctional uterine bleeding, unwanted conception and/or the development of endometrial hyperplasia.
      2) A cyclic progestational agent will regulate menses, but not treat hirsutism. Furthermore, since ovulation may unpredictably and sporadically occur, the risk exists of progestational agent administration in early pregnancy.
      3) Oral contraceptives will suppress pituitary LH and FSH output, prevent ovarian stimulation, with decreased androstenedione and testosterone output, leading to decreased peripheral conversion to estrogens, and suppressed estrogens; contraception is provided and menstrual regulation results. The progression of hirsutism is ordinarily halted.
      4) Corticosteroids have been tried with varying success depending upon the author. Where a significant adrenal component can be diagnosed or suspected, dexamethasone may be appropriate treatment; it is, however, less effective than clomiphene in inducing ovulation. If androgens are successfully suppressed, an improvement in the hirsutism will be observed. However, hirsutism will not diminish at normal circulating androgen levels.
      5) Spironolactone (100-200 mg daily in divided doses) is effective for the treatment of hirsutism as it functions as an antiandrogen at the hair follicle. Effects on androgen levels are variable but improved menstrual cyclicity has been reported. Pregnancy is contraindicated in women taking spironolactone, because of potential demasculinizing effects on fetal male external genitalia. The major side-effect is fatigue, although hyperkalemia has been reported.

"Turned-Off" Hypoestrogenized Chronic Anovulation Syndromes

1. Hypothalamic amenorrhea

   The etiology of the anovulation must be determined.
   Unfortunately, the mechanisms for the several forms of chronic
   anovulation are poorly understood. Hypothalamic anovulation is
   a heterogeneous group of disorders with similar manifestations.
   Anorexia nervosa is the prototype psychogenic and nutritional
   form of amenorrhea and the most severe. There are a group of
   closely related disorders in which emotional stress, diet, body
   composition, exercise, and other unrecognized factors contribute
   in varying proportions to the anovulation.

   A. Anorexia nervosa
      The constellation of amenorrhea which may precede the marked
      weight loss; a bizarre and distorted attitude toward eating,
      food, and body weight; and a distorted body image makes the
      diagnosis of anorexia nervosa obvious in almost all cases.
      It is important, however, not to overlook an organic cause,
      including a hypothalamic lesion.

      Appropriate psychotherapy is the most important therapeutic
      modality. However, forced feeding by gastric tube or
      intravenous hyperalimentation may be required initially in
      severe cases. Behavior modification is now widely used, but
      long-term improvement remains to be determined. Even if
      "recovery" occurs, individuals with anorexia nervosa may
      always have difficulty regulating caloric intake and may
      alternate between obesity and extreme thinness.

   B. Exercise-associated amenorrhea
      Although in many respects affected individuals present
      similarly to those with psychogenic or hypothalamic
      amenorrhea, laboratory data suggest that this group may form
      a distinct entity. Amenorrheic long distance runners
      associated more stress with their running, lost more weight
      with the onset of running, and consumed less of their
      calories as protein than did normal cycling runners. Higher
      basal levels of both LH and DS than commonly seen in other
      forms of this disorder were also observed. A reduction in
      exercise in association with a change in life style is
      effective in inducing resumption of cyclic menses, but most
      athletes find these suggestions unacceptable. Since
      exercise has a positive effect on bone mineralization, most
      amenorrheic exercisers have adequate bone density without
      evidence of osteoporosis. There is no evidence that
      prolonged amenorrhea is harmful, so no therapy is most often

preferred by these women who frequently are pleased by the absence of menses. Clomiphene can be used to induce ovulation in patients desiring pregnancy although patients with extreme hypoestrogenicity may not respond. Factors predisposing female athletes to secondary amenorrhea may include prior menstrual dysfunction or delayed menarche, nulliparity and young age, miles run per week, weight loss, alteration of the percentage of body fat, hyperprolactinemia, increased endorphins, and stress.

C. Stress-associated amenorrhea
This form of anovulation is heterogenous in origin and a common form of amenorrhea. There is a higher incidence of the following factors in these individuals in comparison with a matched control population: unmarried, engaged in "intellectual" occupations, stressful life events, consumption of sedatives and hypnotic drugs, underweight, and previous menstrual irregularities. In our experience, a remarkably high proportion of these patients give a history of psychosexual problems and socioenvironmental trauma, often about the time of puberty.

D. Combined
It is a "rule of thumb" that the combination of two of the above factors is more likely to result in amenorrhea. For example, extreme weight loss (up to 25% body weight) or extended running (50-70 miles/week) must occur for amenorrhea to result, but the combination of mild degrees of weight loss with moderate distance running is frequently associated with amenorrhea.

These data suggest that psychologic counseling and/or a change in the life-style of the individual should be, and frequently are, effective in inducing ovulation. Clomiphene should be regarded as a second alternative and is usually effective in low doses.

2. Pituitary Amenorrhea

Tumor and acquired hypopituitarism are less common than hypothalamic forms of anovulation but must be diagnosed. Serum prolactin is an excellent screening test. Treatment and hormonal replacement therapy must be individualized. Induction of ovulation is generally possible if pregnancy is desired.

3. Gonadal Amenorrhea

Ovarian failure is diagnosed by serial elevated FSH levels; finding three values greater than 50 mIU/ml taken 4 weeks apart

makes this diagnosis. Estrogen replacement should be considered
if this diagnosis is substantiated.

4. Management of "turned-off" (hypoestrogenic) chronic anovulation
   syndromes

   Patients with amenorrhea usually seek care because of concern
   about possible unrecognized significant disease or ill effects
   of the lack of menstruation, desire for menstruation, or desire
   for present or future fertility. The emotional or stressful
   overtones of the problem should be addressed, as attention to
   the etiology may induce a cure. Specific treatable causes
   should receive specific therapy; if weight loss is the cause of
   the amenorrhea, weight gain is a more appropriate therapy than
   ovulation induction or progestin withdrawal.

   Estrogen deficiency in young women should be treated by estrogen
   replacement. In contrast, any patient who has enough
   endometrial proliferation to result in withdrawal bleeding
   should be considered a candidate for cyclic progestin therapy.

   The hypoestrogenism associated with anorectic, runners',
   dancers'and other significantly "turned off" amenorrheas is of
   particular concern because of the possibility of osteoporosis.
   Over 30% of bone mineral has reportedly been lost by some
   patients with anorexia. Bone loss is less in runners because of
   the weight-bearing exercise which provides some degree of
   protection; however, stress fractures are common although it is
   unclear whether these are caused by bone demineralization. Dual
   photon absorptiometry may be useful in some cases to document
   osteoporosis and to be used as a baseline study before estrogen
   replacement therapy in these women.

   Therapy depends upon the etiologic diagnosis, and should be
   appropriate to the patient's chief complaint. If fertility is
   desired, and a serious etiology, or one contraindicating
   pregnancy, is ruled out, then ovulation induction can be
   attempted. If fertility is not an issue, then nothing need be
   done, except that a yearly skull film may be required.
   Obviously, ovulation may occur at any time, and patients not
   specifically interested in fertility who are having unprotected
   intercourse should be provided with a means of contraception.

SUGGESTED READING

Forney JP, Milewich L, Chen GT, et al: Aromatization of
androstenedione to estrone by human adipose tissue in vitro.

Correlation with adipose tissue mass, age, and endometrial neoplasia. J Clin Endocrinol Metabol 53:192, 1981.

Griffing G, Redline R, Jaffee W, Longcope C, Vaitukaitis J: Effect of peripheral sex steroid metabolism on pituitary gonadotropin reserve of women with hypothalamic amenorrhea. Fertil Steril 36:578, 1981.

Loucks AB, Horvath SM: Athletic amenorrhea: A review. Med Sci Sports Exercise 17:56, 1985.

Petrucco OM: Current investigation and therapy of secondary amenorrhoea. Drugs 31:550, 1986.

Sanborn CF, Martin BJ, Wagner Jr WW: Is athletic amenorrhea specific to runners? Am J Obstet Gynecol 143:859, 1982.

Shangold MM: Causes, evaluation, and management of athletic oligo-amenorrhea. Med Clin North Am 69:83, 1985.

Wentz AC, Diamond MP: Weight related amenorrhea. Infertility 9:75, 1986.

Yen SSC: The polycystic ovary syndrome. Clin Endocrinol 12:177, 1980.

Zhang YW, Stern B, Rebar RW: Endocrine comparison of obese menstruating and amenorrheic women. J Clin Endocrinol Metabol 58:1077, 1984.

Chapter 4

Galactorrhea and Hyperprolactinemia

Anne Colston Wentz, M.D.

INTRODUCTION

Galactorrhea and/or hyperprolactinemia in other than the postpartum lactating woman are abnormal; when either is discovered, a systematic approach at diagnosis, evaluation, and therapy is required.

Prolactin, unlike the other protein hormones of the pituitary, is under inhibitory control by prolactin inhibiting factor (PIF) which is probably dopamine. Regulators other than dopamine are also involved in control of prolactin output: for example, gamma-aminobutyric acid (GABA) is a prolactin-inhibiting factor; releasing factors include thyrotropin-releasing hormone (TRH), the endogenous opiates, serotonin, vasoactive intestinal protein (VIP) and perhaps acetylcholine, but the lactotroph will synthesize and release prolactin without specific stimulation whenever released from inhibitory control.

Indications for the measurement of serum prolactin include: (1) ovulatory or menstrual dysfunction, (2) galactorrhea, (3) luteal phase inadequacy, (4) headache, (5) premenstrual tension syndrome, (6) hypothyroidism, and (7) unexplained infertility.

DIFFERENTIAL DIAGNOSIS

From a clinical standpoint, it is important to divide cases of hyperprolactinemia into those which are associated with neoplasm and those which have other non-neoplastic but still pathologic causes. This greatly simplifies the evaluation of the patient who presents either with galactorrhea or hyperprolactinemia.

Hyperprolactinemia is a relatively common finding in women with menstrual dysfunction and reflects derangements of central mechanisms. It was Hippocrates who astutely noted, "If a woman who is not with child, nor has brought forth, have milk, her menses are obstructed."

CAUSES OF HYPERPROLACTINEMIA

I. Physiologic Causes

Pregnancy
Puerperium
Suckling
Breast stimulation

Exercise
Nonspecific stress
Sleep
Meals

II. Drugs and Medications

Pharmacologic neuroleptics
phenothiazines, haloperidol, tricyclic antidepressants,
monoamine oxidase inhibitors, pimozide, sulpiride, clozapine
Anesthetic agents
Sex hormones
estrogen, oral contraceptives, ? progestins
Antihypertensives
reserpine, alpha-methyldopa, clonidine
Histamine receptor antagonists
cimetidine and ranitidine
Opiates
Dopamine antagonists
metoclopramide, domperidone
Other including amphetamines, hallucinogens, verapamil,
alcohol and beer

III. Neoplastic and Non-neoplastic disorders

Brain and Hypothalamic disorders
Destructive and infiltrative: craniopharyngiomas, pineal
tumors, encephalitis, sarcoid, histocytosis X,
eosinophilic granuloma, hemachromatosis, tuberculosis,
metastatic tumor

IV. Pituitary Disorders

Tumors
Growth hormone producing: acromegaly
ACTH producing: Cushing syndrome, Nelson's syndrome
Prolactinomas
Other:
Stalk section or compression, Sheehan's syndrome, empty
sella syndrome, pituitary infarction, pseudotumor cerebri

V. Endocrine

Hypothyroidism
Polycystic ovarian syndrome

DEFINITION OF GALACTORRHEA

The presence of galactorrhea suggests hyperprolactinemia at some time in the patient's history but can be found when prolactin levels are normal. Galactorrhea means the secretion of a milk-like substance from the breast with or without stimulation. Expressible galactorrhea is described in terms of amount, color, and thickness; bloody, green- or brown-colored fluid or pus is not galactorrhea, and should be further evaluated by cytology, culture, and/or mammography. Galactorrhea is characteristically bilateral, and the fluid contains fat globules.

DEFINITION OF HYPERPROLACTINEMIA

An elevated prolactin level should be confirmed. Assays for prolactin vary and prolactin has a pulsatile secretion pattern. Questions to be answered include whether the elevated prolactin level is significant, whether its etiology can be easily explained, and whether it requires further evaluation. A persistently elevated prolactin level should be recognized as an abnormality and the decision made whether further action is needed.

PREVALENCE

The prevalance of galactorrhea in women reportedly ranges from 0.1-32%, and is found in about 12% of parous and 0% of nulliparous women. Of women with galactorrhea, about 90% will have hyperprolactinemia and 34% will have a tumor; of patients with hyperprolactinemia about 50% will have a tumor. In patients with anovulation, galactorrhea, and hyperprolactinemia, approximately 70% will be found to have radiologically diagnosable pituitary tumors.

Only about 10% of patients with galactorrhea will have normal prolactin levels, and almost none will have a pituitary tumor. Etiologic causes of galactorrhea with normal prolactin levels include:

1. Postpartum
2. Breast stimulation: chronic abscess, manipulation
3. Chest wall lesions: herpes zoster, mastectomy, other side, thoracotomy, burns
4. Spinal cord lesions: tabes, syringomyelia

CLINICAL MANIFESTATIONS

Galactorrhea is the clinical manifestation of hyperprolactinemia. A drop of breast discharge can be put on a glass slide, smeared for cytology if indicated and a Sudan B fat stain used to indicate the presence of fat, which suggests hyperprolactinemia; in the absence of the stain, fat globules are easily observed under the light microscope. Patients presenting with galactorrhea may or may not have elevated prolactin levels.

In taking the history in a patient with galactorrhea, determine if ever the patient had any reason to have an elevated prolactin; a history of pregnancy, taking oral contraceptives or other estrogen-containing medications, or phenothiazine use are all associated with secondary hyperprolactinemia. With past hyperprolactinemia, galactorrhea is less likely to be a manifestation of primary hyperprolactinemia which might be due to a pituitary adenoma. On the other hand, when initially evaluating a patient for galactorrhea who claims no etiologic reason for an elevated prolactin level, then this patient should be very carefully evaluated for the possibility of an adenoma.

Menstrual abnormalities occur in 80-90%, and amenorrhea in 50-75% of women with galactorrhea. Hypogonadism may be observed. However, 50% of women demonstrated to have galactorrhea did not know of the discharge. Galactorrhea due to a central cause may be unilateral, although a unilateral breast discharge is more often associated with a problem localized in the breast.

EVALUATION

Initial Evaluation

1. History: Ask about medications, look for pharmacologic causes; determine when galactorrhea developed, with or without an obviously elevated prolactin level; has the patient been pregnant, had chest surgery, head injury, or neurologic symptoms
2. Physical: Check reflexes (hypothyroidism)
3. Pelvic examination places the patient, if amenorrheic, in either the "turned-on" or "turned-off" classification (see Chapter 3)
4. Laboratory Work-up
   a. Pregnancy test
   b. Repeat prolactin
   c. TSH, T_4

After history, physical, and pelvic examination, certain laboratory tests are essential. All patients with galactorrhea require prolactin levels, and every patient with an elevated prolactin level requires serum TSH, looking for hypothyroidism. Further evaluation depends upon the patient's presentation, and might include gonadotropins in most amenorrheic patients, and measurement of androgens in those with hirsutism.

Further Evaluation

1. CT scan of the sella turcica, with coronal and sagittal views with and without contrast should be considered in any patient with hyperprolactinemia; a CT scan is definitely indicated when: (a) the prolactin level is twice the upper limit of normal for the assay used in patients without a history of taking prolactin-increasing drugs; and (b) definitely indicated when the patient wants pregnancy.

2. Visual fields should be obtained (a) for baseline evaluation in any patient with hyperprolactinemia and a microadenoma before pregnancy; (b) are indicated in any patient with macroadenoma, and; (c) should be repeated every 4 weeks during pregnancy in any patient with a macroadenoma (tumor size 1.0 cm or greater).

We have done CT scans routinely in virtually all patients with hyperprolactinemia. The use of a coned-down x-ray of the sella turcica reveals only large tumors, and hypocycloidal tomography has an unacceptable false-negative and false-positive rate. CT scanning will diagnose the empty sella syndrome, craniopharyngioma, and other hypothalamic entities impinging upon pituitary function. Magnetic resonance imaging (MRI) is a new technique which has the advantage of no radiation exposure and, therefore, can be used during pregnancy. Resolution is a problem (at this writing) so the technique has limits in defining small (less than 1 cm) pituitary lesions; MRI is, however, anticipated to replace CT scanning.

Dynamic pituitary testing has been of little diagnostic value in our hands. The use of a TRH stimulation has not been helpful in delineating the patients with prolactinomas. Insulin tolerance tests and stimulation with hypothalamic releasing factors give a hormonal profile of the patient but add little to clinical management.

When a pituitary tumor is found, a screen for normal pituitary function in terms of other hormone output may be indicated. A macroadenoma with only moderate hyperprolactinemia may suggest hyperfunction of another pituitary cell type. Draw TSH (if not done previously), ACTH and/or cortisol, growth hormone or somatomedin-C levels. Consider utilizing dynamic pituitary testing with hypothalamic factors, a glucose tolerance test to evalute a paradoxical growth hormone increase, and insulin tolerance testing to check for hypofunction.

MANAGEMENT OF HYPERPROLACTINEMIA SYNDROMES

GOALS OF THERAPY

Reverse signs and symptoms of tumor mass effect
Prevent development or growth of tumor
Preserve hormone function
Correct symptoms
Restore fertility
Stop galactorrhea
Restore normal menstruation
Restore libido and potency
Prevent decreased bone mineral content

As always, the chief complaint of the patient dictates to a major extent the therapeutic approach. The patient's expectations must be balanced with numerous variables which include: the etiology of the hyperprolactinemia; the presence or absence of pituitary tumor; its size; desire for fertility; age of the patient; an assessment of risk factors, including increased tumor size and osteoporosis; and the motivation or compliance of the patient. There are numerous goals of therapy and several alternative approaches to achieve these goals.

THERAPEUTIC OPTIONS IN HYPERPROLACTINEMIA

1. Dopamine agonists
     Parlodel
     Pergolide
2. Surgery
     Transsphenoidal resection
     Craniotomy
3. Radiation
4. Observation
5. ? GnRH analogues

1. Dopamine agonists

Parlodel is an ergot alkaloid dopamine agonist which rapidly suppresses prolactin levels by inhibiting the release of prolactin,

which subsequently results in a shut-down in synthesis of the
hormone.

Pergolide mesylate is a long-acting dopamine agonist that binds
to dopamine receptors on pituitary lactotrophs, inhibits prolactin
production, and reduces serum prolactin in normal individuals as
well as those with hyperprolactinemia. This drug is not presently
available, although effective, with relatively mild side-effects.

Parlodel may be started at a relatively low dose, either 1.25
or 2.5 mg, and given only at bedtime to minimize the minimal side
effects, which include postural hypotension, headaches, and nausea.
Once past the initial phase of administration, most patients can
tolerate an increased dosage without side-effects. On the other
hand, the administration of too large a dose from the outset, for
example, 7.5 mg daily as recommended for the treatment of postpartum
patients to suppress lactation, is associated with side-effects in
almost 100% of patients, and will make virtually all of them
discontinue the medication.

Parlodel administration is associated with a reduction of
prolactin levels to normal within days and a rapid decrease in
galactorrhea within weeks. Ordinarily, a return to near normal
prolactin levels is necessary for the patient to resume ovulatory
function; since this may occur quite rapidly, the patient must be
cautioned about the rapid return of ovulation, and barrier
contraception is prescribed as required.

In patients wanting pregnancy, a cycle or more before
discontinuing contraception is advisable to restore hormonal
balances and replete estrogen-derived tissues. In patients not
wanting pregnancy, contraception may be problematic since
estrogen-containing oral contraceptives are probably
contraindicated.

In patients with visual field defects during pregnancy,
Parlodel administration, 7.5 or 10 mg daily, rapidly reverts the
field changes to normal. Since tumor expansion will recur quickly
with discontinuation of medical treatment, once Parlodel is
instituted during pregnancy, it should be continued. Breast-feeding
is not contraindicated in these patients, and the risk of tumor
expansion is less because of the lower estradiol levels postpartum.
Parlodel is not cleared for usage during pregnancy, but no
congenital defects have been reported associated with its
administration. However, patients are cautioned to discontinue the
drug when pregnancy is diagnosed.

2. Surgery

The surgical approach for the treatment of prolactinomas is
ordinarily reserved for patients with macroadenomas greater than 10
mm; although smaller tumors can clearly be removed with ease (49-81%
complete removal for the microadenomas and 19-40% for
macroadenomas), in the microadenoma group, most revert to
hyperprolactinemia within a year after surgery. Since
transsphenoidal adenectomy is usually not associated with cure,
surgery is usually recommended for the largest tumors or perhaps for
patients with tumors resistant to bromocriptine treatment. These
would include patients previously treated with bromocriptine who had
either no significant reduction or even a progressive increase in
adenoma size, who failed to achieve adequate reduction of serum
prolactin, who have complaints about the inconvenience of high daily
dosages or side effects, and who cannot afford the cost of chronic
medical therapy. In bromocriptine pretreated patients, the rate of
successful surgical outcome is not significantly different from that
of patients without presurgical pharmacotherapy. The lactotrophs
treated with bromocriptine undergo considerable fibrosis which
accounts for a more difficult operation and perhaps the lack of
difference in results.

In general, transsphenoidal resection results in a 70-80%
chance of decrease in prolactin concentration; measurement of
prolactin prior to the patient's discharge from the hospital is
prognostic with respect to resumption of ovulatory menstrual
function, and to return of tumor growth. The size of the tumor
clearly influences the completeness of its removal, but
transsphenoidal resection is unlikely to provide a permanent cure in
most patients operated. Although the surgery is relatively safe,
postoperative diabetes insipidus occurs in greater than 60% of
patients; sinusitis, rhinitis, and meningitis are also reported.
Approximately 50% of tumors recur in the 3-5 years after surgery.
For this reason, transsphenoidal surgery is now reserved for those
patients with enlarging lesions, and for those with macroadenomas
who desire pregnancy.

3. Radiation

Proton beam therapy is effective for midline lesions, but is
available in very few centers in the United States. Other forms of
radiotherapy are less successful, because prolactin-producing tumors
are not particularly radiosensitive. Yttrium 90 implants have been
used, but this technique can be complicated by optic neuritis,
dislodging of the Yttrium implant, hypopituitarism, and diabetes
insipidus.

4. Observation

Some patients with prolactin producing microadenomoas, particularly those not interested in or at risk for pregnancy, need little other than observation, as their risk factors appear to be minimal. In the absence of significant hypoestrogenism, very high prolactin levels, osteopenia and complete amenorrhea, then observation may be indicated. A prolactin drawn yearly is indicated, and some patients may need to be followed with CT scans.

The routine follow-up of patients with minimal hyperprolactinemia and small tumors may also include the use of MRI as with this technique, radiation dosage is minimized. Although available in only a few centers at present, it nevertheless will become widely available. Once sufficient resolution has been achieved, MRI will become the method of choice for the follow-up of these tumors.

5. GnRH Analogues

GnRH, which stimulates the output of both FSH and LH, has also been found to increase the output of prolactin. The mechanism is probably by a paracrine effect. Since the continuous administration of GnRH will decrease pituitary FSH and LH output by a "down-regulation" mechanism, and since GnRH analogues are even more potent in suppressing pituitary secretion, it has been suggested that the use of suppressive GnRH analogues may have an effect upon lactotroph prolactin production. Although untested at present, the possibility of the use of gonadotropin releasing hormone analogues should be followed.

PATIENT MANAGEMENT

Patients interested in pregnancy: The desire for fertility becomes the major dividing line in deciding therapeutic options for patients with hyperprolactinemia. Patients interested in pregnancy should use a barrier method of contraception until the etiology of the hyperprolactinemia has been evaluated, contraindications to ovulation induction and pregnancy eliminated, and an ovulatory cycle re-established.

Patients with hyperprolactinemia and pituitary adenomas less than 10 mm will usually respond to administration of Parlodel. The ideal drug for medical treatment should have rapid action, be free of side-effects, safe, effective and inexpensive; Parlodel comes close to achieving these goals.

Parlodel dosage: Gradually increasing Parlodel dosage to achieve significant suppression of prolactin is well tolerated by most patients. Parlodel, 1.25 mg at bedtime for 7 days, followed by 2.5 mg at bedtime for 2 weeks, with reassessment of prolactin levels, and an increase in dosage as required will work for most patients without inducing nausea, hypotension, and other side-effects. Keeping a basal temperature chart is useful to assess return of ovulatory function. Usually, little ovarian response in terms of estrogen output or follicular development is observed until prolactin levels have returned close to the normal range. With persistant hyperprolactinemia, luteal phase inadequacy may be diagnosed. Less than 10% of patients require a dosage in excess of 10 mg/day, and most patients can be maintained satisfactorily on 5 mg daily.

Once an ovulatory cycle has occurred, the barrier method of contraception may be discontinued to permit attempts at pregnancy. If pregnancy does not occur within three cycles, then further evaluation of the adequacy of hormonal output, tubal function and male factor are indicated.

Once pregnancy is diagnosed, Parlodel is discontinued. No increase in congenital anomalies due to the drug has been reported, but Parlodel has not been cleared for use in pregnancy. Further, discontinuing the drug with onset of pregnancy allows it to be reinstituted should problems with the pregnancy occur.

The Anticipated Effects of Bromocriptine Therapy
(in microadenoma patients)

Normalized PRL	95%
Reduced tumor size	80%
Restored fertility	60-70%
Normalized visual fields	62%
Restored pituitary function	60%

Management of pregnancy: Measurement of serum prolactin is prognostically useless in pregnancy. CT scanning provides too great a radiation exposure. MRI may be useful, but is not widely available for clinical purposes.

Baseline visual field testing is recommended before pregnancy is attempted, and monthly during pregnancy, with more frequent evaluation should symptomatology such as headaches occur. Reinstitution of Parlodel is indicated if visual field abnormalities are detected, and these field cuts usually resolve without incident.

Patients not desiring fertility: Patients with hyperprolactinemia who are ovulating and menstruating relatively normally do not ordinarily require Parlodel; the immunologically active prolactin measured may not be biologically active.

Amenorrheic patients must be assessed on the basis of their other findings. Prolactin affects bone, and may exacerbate bone demineralization. In thin, nonexercising women with significant hyperprolactinemia, ovarian estradiol output may be quite low, with resultant osteoporosis. These women should be treated with Parlodel and not estrogen, because estrogen is stimulatory to the lactotroph and increases prolactin secretion. However, well-estrogenized amenorrheic patients with hyperprolactinemia ordinarily do not require suppressive treatment, and probably should be cycled using a progestational agent for endometrial protection.

Management of patients with macroadenomas: The transsphenoidal approach to the surgical removal of prolactin adenomas is ordinarily satisfactory, but far more difficult with larger tumors. A surgical approach is recommended in patients with large tumors, or those in whom the response to bromocriptine has been inconsistent or complicated by side-effects. If the tissue diagnosis is at all in doubt, a surgical approach may be indicated, particularly where the possibility of an intrasellar craniopharyngioma is suspected.

FACTORS PREDICTIVE OF SURGICAL SUCCESS

Size of tumor	< 1 cm
Production level	< 200 ng/ml
Sex	Female
Age	18-26 years
Duration of amenorrhea	< 6 years
Estrogen-related onset	

Natural history: Hyperprolactinemia, due either to micro/or macroadenomas is usually a long-term problem.

PROBLEMS OF PROLACTINOMAS

Lifelong therapy
Unknown long-term effects
With discontinuation of therapy:
    Resumption of hyperprolactinemia
    Resumption of tumor growth

For, these reasons, patients should be educated not with alarm but for informational purposes about future management, risk factors, and symptoms of sufficient concern (dry vagina, hypoestrogenism, headaches, visual problems) to report.

SUGGESTED READING

Andersen AN: Hyperprolactinemia - Influence on hypothalamic-pituitary-gonadal axis. Danish Med Bull 31:413, 1984.

Grossman A, Besser GM: Prolactinomas. Br Med J 290:182, 1985.

Judd SJ: Primary hyperprolactinaemia and chronic anovulation: Pathophysiology and management. Clin Reprod Fertil 1:95, 1982.

Koppelman MCS, Jaffe MJ, Rieth KG, Caruso RC, Loriaux DL: Hyperprolactinemia, amenorrhea, and galactorrhea. Ann Int Med 100:115, 1984.

Pepperell RJ: Prolactin and reproduction. Fertil Steril 35:267, 1981.

Sakiyama R, Quan M: Galactorrhea and hyperprolactinemia. Obstet Gynecol Surv 38:689, 1983.

Strauch G: Which treatment for hyperprolactinemic females? Hormone Res 22:215, 1985.

Chapter 5

Oligomenorrhea and Abnormal Uterine Bleeding

Anne Colston Wentz, M.D.

DEFINITION

A. Bleeding abnormal in DURATION, AMOUNT, or FREQUENCY for a particular patient.

Vaginal bleeding which is abnormal in duration, frequency, or amount deserves evaluation. This is the abnormality which brings the patient to the doctor, and which needs correction. The evaluation establishes the source of the bleeding, which is usually the uterus. Abnormal uterine bleeding is to be distinguished from dysfunctional uterine bleeding (DUB). DUB is usually defined as abnormal bleeding for which no organic cause can be found by the usual techniques of history, physical and pelvic examination. The etiology usually is a disturbance of hormonal function, and a lack of uterine pathology is implied; however, uterine myomata, endometrial polyps and even malignancy may ultimately be diagnosed, which suggests that DUB is a diagnosis of exclusion which can only be made by an extensive evaluation. Therefore, for the purposes of detailing a logical and effective approach, we start with the abnormality which brings the patient to the doctor, which is bleeding considered to be abnormal in duration, frequency or amount, and describe the steps in diagnosis and evaluation which lead to successful management.

B. Patterns of bleeding

Normal menstruation: Flow lasting 3-8 days, blood loss 30-80 ml, cycle length 30 ± 4 days.

Oligomenorrhea: Infrequent, irregular episodes of bleeding, occurring at intervals greater than 40 days.

Polymenorrhea: Frequent, but regular episodes of uterine
                bleeding, usually occurring at intervals
                of 21 days or less.

Hypermenorrhea: Uterine bleeding excessive in both amount
  (Menorrhagia) and duration of flow, occurring at regular
                 intervals.

Metrorrhagia: Uterine bleeding, usually not excessive,
               occurring at irregular intervals.

Menometrorrhagia: Uterine bleeding, usually excessive and
                   prolonged occurring at frequent and
                   irregular intervals.

Hypomenorrhea: Uterine bleeding that is regular, but
                decreased in amount.

Intermenstrual Uterine bleeding, usually not excessive,
  bleeding: occurring between otherwise regular
                menstrual periods.

EVALUATION OF ABNORMAL UTERINE BLEEDING

A. History
B. Physical and pelvic examinations
C. Endometrial biopsy
D. Laboratory evaluation

Abnormal uterine bleeding (AUB) is a symptom and not a
diagnosis. The therapy of AUB must be based on etiologic diagnosis.
Diagnosis is approached by a systematic consideration of those
central, intermediate, and peripheral entities which can be
associated with abnormal bleeding.

Exogenous hormones are frequently used in the therapy of DUB.
A primary concern of this chapter is to make the point that hormonal
treatment must be based on an etiologic diagnosis of the bleeding.

The history should detail the bleeding abnormality, and attempt
to ascertain if the patient is or is not ovulatory. Does bleeding
occur in regular or irregular intervals, what is the span or
duration, and is it predictable? When does bleeding occur, and how
much blood is lost? This can be estimated from the number of pads
or tampons used, the presence or absence of clots and the duration
of menses. It is also useful to ask about cramps and other

associated pain, and the degree to which the bleeding interferes
with active life. Describe, qualitate and quantitate. Set the
setting in which the bleeding occurs.

The physical examination must exclude intermediate factors such
as chronic and debilitating disease, and obvious endocrinopathies.

Pelvic examination must exclude obvious organic causes of
bleeding (vaginitis, Trichomonas, cervical polyps, ectropion,
cervical carcinoma, foreign bodies, myomata uteri, incomplete
abortion, ovarian enlargement).

Laboratory Evaluation. The patient with AUB should have
certain tests performed:

1. Endometrial biopsy should be performed on the initial visit
   if the patient is bleeding. Tell the patient to make an
   appointment to be seen for a biopsy immediately if bleeding
   occurs.

2. Complete hematologic work-up with platelet count to rule out
   blood dyscrasias should be done.

3. Hormone studies, particularly in the anovulatory patient;
   FSH, LH, androgen levels (testosterone and DS) and a
   prolactin level are most useful in establishing an etiologic
   diagnosis.

4. Thyroid function tests should be considered although the
   yield will be low. Patients with sufficient thyroid
   dysfunction to have AUB should be obvious on physical
   examination.

MANAGEMENT GOALS

A. Arrest of the acute bleeding episode

For the patient who presents bleeding heavily, an approach is
needed which controls the blood loss and arrives quickly at a
diagnosis. The most common causes must be kept in mind. Virtually
every patient with profuse bleeding not due to cancer or pregnancy
will respond to a vigorous endometrial biopsy, using wall suction or
syringe suction, followed by the administration of intramuscular
progesterone. The tissue obtained will make the diagnosis, and this
can be immediate if a frozen section is available.

1. Most common causes
   Cancer
   Pregnancy complication
   Anovulatory AUB
   Submucous myoma

2. Treatment
   a. curettage (if bleeding is exceedingly heavy)
   b. office suction biopsy (is usually sufficient)
   c. progesterone 100-200 mg IM repeated in 4-6 hours if necessary
   d. oral progestational agent for 7-10 days, beginning immediately
      1. Norlutin 5-10 mg BID
      2. Provera 10-20 mg BID

The vast majority of patients stop bleeding within 24-36 hours with this approach. Intravenous estrogen is not needed, and is contraindicated in the patient whose bleeding is from a hyperplastic endometrium. If the patient does not respond, then a blood dyscrasia or a submucous myoma should be ruled out. A thorough hematologic evaluation and an ultrasound examination are indicated.

Usually, however, the vaginal bleeding is not catastrophic, and the etiologic diagnosis can be readily established. No attempt to stop light bleeding is usually needed, until diagnosis-directed therapy can be instituted.

B. Prevention of recurrence, restoration of cyclic menses

   1. establish the diagnosis
      endometrial biopsy during bleeding is useful for diagnosis
   2. find and treat the etiology

An important principle is to think ahead to future management. It is insufficient simply to make the diagnosis as bleeding may recur. "Restoration of cyclic menses" implies an end result of regular, predictable bleeding, which may be accomplished by restoring the patient's own ovulatory cyclicity, by treating with oral contraceptives to achieve cyclic bleeding or by instituting cyclic withdrawal bleeding using a progestational agent for the first 10-14 days of each month.

DIFFERENTIAL DIAGNOSIS

A. First step: determine the source of the bleeding
    1. Cervical
        a. neoplastic problems, including polyps, carcinoma
        b. cervical erosions, eversions, cervicitis
        c. cervical condylomata
    2. Vaginal
        a. carcinoma or adenosis
        b. laceration or injury from coitus or attempts at
            abortion
        c. foreign bodies, including pessaries
        d. local infections, including Trichomonas
            (strawberry patches)
    3. Bleeding from other sites
        a. urethra, urinary tract
        b. rectum, gastrointestinal tract
        c. external genitalia
            1) labial trauma, inflammation, condylomata,
               varices
            2) neoplasia
            3) infectious disease, including viral

B. Next, consider and specifically rule out:
    1. Complications of a past pregnancy
    2. Threatened or incomplete abortion
    3. Ectopic pregnancy
    4. Organic pelvic disease
        a. neoplastic
        b. infectious (tuberculosis, granulomatous
            endometritis, pelvic inflammatory disease)

C. And finally: determine the etiology. Begin by first deciding
    whether the bleeding is ovulatory or anovulatory.

    1. Ovulatory Abnormal Uterine Bleeding

        A. Types of abnormal uterine bleeding associated with
            ovulatory cycles
            1. Bleeding at ovulation
            2. Polymenorrhea due to follicular shortening, or
                to luteal shortening
            3. Irregular endometrial shedding, including
                premenstrual staining, prolonged menses
            4. Persistent corpus luteum (Halban's disease)
            5. Blood dyscrasias, such as ITP, von
                Willebrand's disease, leukemia

6. Iatrogenic, including drugs such as anticoagulants, progestational agents, intrauterine devices and contraceptives.
7. Complications of a past pregnancy, including retained secundines, placental polyps
8. Ectopic pregnancy
9. Organic pelvic disease, including neoplastic disease (benign or malignant), infectious diseases, endometriosis, adenomyosis

Bleeding at ovulation is usually scant, lasting 2-3 days. Endometrial biopsy shows either late proliferative, interval, or early secretory endometrium. The bleeding may be due to rupture of the follicle with fimbrial pick-up of blood. Circulating E_2 levels decrease at the time of the LH surge, and the abrupt fall may interrupt endometrial integrity.

Treatment is usually not necessary. Consider doing a D & C if the bleeding represents a significant problem.

Polymenorrhea, usually implies an 18 to 21-day cycle. Either follicular phase shortening, or luteal phase shortening, is shown by evaluation of basal body temperature chart and endometrial biopsy.

Treatment: For follicular shortening, Premarin 0.3-0.6 mg, days 3-10 is usually effective.
For luteal phase shortening, progesterone suppositories, 25 mg twice daily from 2 days after ovulation, are an effective but unusual treatment and primarily reserved for the patient with infertility. Provera and other progestational agents cannot be used without a method of contraception.
Oral contraceptives provide an approach to the therapy of this particular type of bleeding if the diagnosis is first documented.

Irregular shedding is characterized by prolonged and profuse bleeding at regular intervals. An endometrial biopsy taken at least 5 days after the onset of menses will show a variable pattern including secretory endometrium, incomplete regeneration, and some proliferative tissue. This may indicate retarded regression of the corpus luteum.

Treatment: Curettage is usually effective.
Premarin, 0.6-1.25 mg, days 2-6.
Oral contraceptives

Premenstrual staining may be due to endometriosis and/or
adenomyosis, or to a submucous myoma covered with a thin and poorly
supported endometrium. Endometrial biopsy will usually show a
glandular-stromal disparity, including inadequate perivascular
cuffing and poor decidual formation. Chronic endometritis may be
seen with a submucous myoma.

Treatment: Progesterone or a progestational agent can be given
on days 20-25; oral contraceptives are frequently
effective.

Hypermenorrhea or menorrhagia is very often due to organic
causes, including blood dyscrasias, myomata uteri, polyps and the
like. A D & C should be performed either just before or with the
bleeding. Treatment is based on the etiologic diagnosis, but the
hypermenorrhea will usually respond to oral contraceptives, or such
progestational agents as Norlutin or Provera given for at least 20
days. An unusual cause of hypermenorrhea may be adenomyosis.
Methergine, 0.2 mg BID-QID, as a therapeutic trial during menses may
be useful; the diagnosis is difficult to make, although a
symmetrically-enlarged, boggy uterus may be palpated. The
administration of progestational drugs or androgens is ordinarily
not useful, and curettage is neither diagnostic nor therapeutic.

The persistent corpus luteum, Halban's disease, does not
usually recur in cyclic fashion. Endometrial biopsy may show
secretory endometrium or glandular-stromal disparity. Diagnosis is
difficult but best made by observing a prolonged luteal phase on
basal temperature chart, relatively non-tender, unilateral ovarian
enlargement, and a negative sensitive pregnancy test. An ectopic
pregnancy must be considered and carefully ruled out. A decidual
cast is sometimes passed in either condition.

Blood dyscrasias, rarely causing AUB, are diagnosed by
appropriate hematologic studies. Long-term suppression of menses in
severe anemias may be accomplished by progestational agents, such as
continuous Norlutin or injectable Depo-Provera.

2.   Anovulatory Abnormal Uterine Bleeding

    A.   Types of abnormal uterine bleeding associated with anovulation
        1.   Central hypothalamic/pituitary causes
            a.   Functional and organic disease, including traumatic, toxic, and infectious lesions
            b.   psychogenic factors including stress, anxiety, emotional trauma
            c.   Neurogenic factors, including pituitary tumors
        2.   Intermediate causes, such as chronic illness, metabolic or endocrine disease and nutritional disturbances
        3.   Peripheral causes, including ovarian cysts and tumors and premature ovarian failure

The etiology of anovulatory AUB is approached by consideration of those central, intermediate, and peripheral factors associated with anovulation. Anovulatory bleeding may be heavy or light, constant or intermittent, and rarely may be exsanguinating. The bleeding is usually not associated with symptoms of premenstrual tension, irritability, fluid shift, or cramps, although the patient who passes large clots may have a painful episode. Characteristically, a period of amenorrhea is followed by 10-14 days of profuse bleeding, and a week or more of spotting.

The endometrial biopsy during bleeding may be proliferative or hyperplastic, indicating unopposed estrogen stimulation. A typical hormonal pattern is seen, with elevated LH and normal FSH, and elevated androgen levels. E_2 levels may be low, while estrone is usually elevated. A D & C may be needed, but does nothing to prevent a future occurrence. Physicians tend to forget that a D & C is therapy only for the present episode, and is rarely curative except in the presence of organic pathology. Preventive medicine should be practiced if anovulatory bleeding is diagnosed.

Patients with AUB show different types of hormonal patterns, depending somewhat on the time of life, and management varies with pattern.

The pubertal patient with abnormal bleeding is usually just beginning to establish an ovulatory cycle, and may have various abnormalities of hormonal output; an inadequate FSH output, inadequate LH surge, and inadequate LH maintenance of the luteal phase have all been documented. Most often, the interval between bleeding is increased, and rarely is menstruation profuse. As maturation occurs, the periods become more regular.

Treatment: The best treatment for this group of patients is no treatment at all. Reassurance is essential, but usually time, with attendant maturation, will cure the problem. The rare patient with profuse bleeding may occasionally require hormonal treatment; several cycles with an oral contraceptive may reassure such a patient that menstruation can be predictable and manageable. Alternatively, 3 or 4 months of Norlutin, 5 mg daily for 25 days, beginning on cycle day 5, will usually suffice.

The reproductive age abnormal bleeder most often has a polycystic ovarian syndrome, with chronic anovulation, a relative increase in LH over FSH values, and a failure of the LH surge. These patients tend to be both hyperandrogenic and hyperestrogenic.

Treatment: Treatment of anovulatory bleeding in the reproductive age group is based upon the chief complaint of the patient. The physician and patient have four alternative approaches in management:

1. ovulation induction, ordinarily clomiphene citrate
2. oral contraceptives
3. cyclic progestational agents, if a barrier method of contraception is used
4. observation

If fertility is desired, induction of ovulation will usually cure the abnormal bleeding. The reader is referred to the section on ovulation induction.

If fertility is not an issue, but the bleeding is profuse and troubling, care and concern are essential in the management. Ovarian estrogen output is usually increased in these patients, and a hyperplastic endometrium may develop. The unopposed estrogen stimulation, therefore, should be interrupted periodically. This may be accomplished by:

Provera, 10 mg p.o. for the first 10-12 days of each month
Norlutin, 5 mg p.o. for 10-12 days
Micronor, 2 mg for the first 12 days of each month

Taking the drug orally for the first 10-12 days of each month by the calendar is convenient and easily remembered. However, the progestational agents are not contraceptives and irregular ovulation may occur unpredictably. A barrier method of contraception should be used.

The oral contraceptives provide suppression of ovulation and regular periods. They will effectively suppress FSH and LH output, increase testosterone-binding globulin, and result in decreased circulating testosterone; this is advantageous for the majority of reproductive age patients with AUB who probably have a form of polycystic ovaries.

The diagnosis of atypical endometrial hyperplasia obtained on an endometrial biopsy necessitates the performance of a D & C. The degree of atypia discovered dictates further management. With mild atypical hyperplasia, either treatment with a progestational agent or ovulation induction, may be curative; follow-up is obviously needed. With moderate or worse atypical hyperplasia, long-term suppression with progestational agents may be attempted especially in younger patients in whom fertility is an issue. Megace, 40 mg daily for 3 months, has been successful. An atrophic or proliferative endometrium on biopsy after 3 months therapy suggests an adequate response. However, a D & C must be repeated 4-6 weeks later to document this, and a plan, either to induce ovulation, or to cycle using a progestational agent must be instituted to prevent a recurrence.

The anovulatory dysfunctional bleeder, characteristically obese, hypertensive, and latently diabetic, is at obvious risk for the development of endometrial adenocarcinoma. Three episodes of profuse and troubling bleeding, necessitating transfusion, should suggest consideration of hysterectomy if child-bearing has been accomplished.

If fertility is not an issue, and the bleeding simply irregular but not profuse or of concern, then observation is appropriate and nothing need be done except to explain to the patient that regular clinic visits must be made. These patients usually do not have sufficient unopposed estrogen to develop a hyperplastic endometrium. They usually ovulate irregularly and should be told that conception may occur.

The perimenopausal pattern of dysfunctional bleeding is primarily related to impending ovarian failure. FSH values tend to be elevated while LH values remain within the normal menstrual limits. The perimenopausal patient has a characteristic pattern, with gradually lengthening intervals between bleeding. Sporadic and less frequent ovulation occurs, and ultimately, menopause intervenes.

Treatment: D & C is essential in the perimenopausal woman with abnormal bleeding, and is frequently curative. As in the pubertal patient, the passage of time may permit resolution of the problem.

Again, Provera, 10 mg, or Norlutin, 5 mg, for 10-12 days every 4-6 weeks to induce endometrial shedding will usually suffice. It should be remembered that the primary etiologic cause of abnormal bleeding in the perimenopausal patient is estrogen administration. Intractable and profuse bleeding necessitates hysterectomy.

SUMMARY

1. Establish source of bleeding to be uterine
2. Establish whether the bleeding is:
   Acute or chronic
   Ovulatory or anovulatory
3. Make a definitive etiologic diagnosis
4. Re-establish menstrual cyclicity and prevent recurrence

SUGGESTED READING

Aksel S, Jones GS: Etiology and treatment of dysfunctional uterine bleeding. Obstet Gynecol 44:1-13, 1974.

Claessens EA, Cowell CA: Acute adolescent menorrhagia. Am J Obstet Gynecol 139:277-280, 1981.

Davies AJ, Anderson ABM, Turnbull AC: Reduction by Naproxen of excessive menstrual bleeding in women using intrauterine devices. Obstet Gynecol 57:74-78, 1981.

Goldfarb JM, Little AB: Current concepts. N Engl J Med 302:666-669, 1980.

Lidor A, Ismajovich B, Confino E, David MP: Histopathological findings in 226 women with post-menopausal uterine bleeding. Acta Obstet Gynecol Scand 65:41, 1986.

Makarainen L, Ylikorkala O: Ibuprofen prevents IUCD-induced increases in menstrual blood loss. Br J Obstet Gynaecol 93:285, 1986.

van Bogaert LJ: Diagnostic aid of endometrium biopsy. Gynecol Obstet Invest 10:289-297, 1979.

Wentz AC: Abnormal uterine bleeding. Primary Care 3:9-22, 1976.

Ylikorkala O, Pekonen F: Naproxen reduces idiopathic but not fibromyoma-induced menorrhagia. Obstet Gynecol 68:10, 1986.

Chapter 6

Diagnosis and Treatment of Hirsutism

Carl M. Herbert III, M.D.

An approach to the evaluation and management of patients complaining of hirsutism requires a basic knowledge of the physiology of hair growth and an understanding of the differences between hypertrichosis, hirsutism, and virilization.

There are three types of hairs:

1. Lanugo - soft fetal hair primarily under the control of growth hormone and shed at 7-8 months gestation.

2. Vellus - thin, nonpigmented, nonmedullated hair also stimulated by growth hormone.

3. Terminal - Course, curly, medullated, pigmented hair, also known as sexual hair.

Transformation from vellus to terminal hair is an androgen dependent process. The sensitivity of this transformation depends upon the site on the body and the racial or genetic background of the individual involved. The most sensitive areas of the body for this transformation are the axillary and pubic areas followed in order by the upper lip, lower abdomen, chin, chest, and lower back. Once vellus to terminal hair transformation has occurred, lower androgen levels can maintain terminal hair growth than those required for the original transformation process.

The hair growth cycle has three phases:

1. Anagen - the phase of active growth

2. Catagen - a transitional involution phase

3. Telogen - the resting phase during which hairs are shed as a result of trauma and by the reactivation of growth within the follicle.

Hair follicles have different cycles of activity depending on their body location. For example, scalp hair follicles normally rest for 3 months and are active for 2-6 years. Facial hair in the male has a similar cycle to the scalp. However, eye brows and eyelashes complete a cycle in less than a year.

Hair growth patterns can be divided into these categories:

I. Asexual Patterns - found in scalp hair, eyebrows, and eyelashes which is present in most individuals regardless of sex or age.

II. Terminal Patterns

A. Ambisexual - pubic and axillary hair stimulated by androgens regardless of sex.

B. Sexual - male hair distribution including beard, chest, abdomen, and sacral areas.

In women, ambisexual hair patterns are observed when androgen levels are within normal limits for females. However, elevated androgens stimulate hair growth in a male distribution. The differences in distribution and amount of terminal hair in the male and female are primarily due to the levels of circulating androgens. Males and females have similar numbers of hair follicles at birth and no new hair follicles appear thereafter. There is some amount of hair follicle loss with increasing age.

Hypertrichosis describes excessive growth of vellus hair. This growth is generally in a nonsexual hair distribution such as over the lumbar spine or the back of the arms. Localized hypertrichosis may be due to trauma or chronic inflammation, steroid application, pretibial myxedema, and nevi or congenital anomalies, e.g. spina bifida occulta. Generalized hypertrichosis may be observed with anorexia nervosa, hypothyroidism, porphyria, and certain nervous system disorders. Hirsutism, on the other hand, defines vellus-terminal hair transformation, usually due to excess androgen stimulation, resulting in an excessive growth of terminal hair in a male distribution. Virilism generally represents a more severe form of hyperandrogenism. In this condition, hirsutism is found in conjunction with a complex of other symptoms including temporal balding, acne, deepening of the voice, decrease in breast size, increase in muscle mass, and/or clitoromegaly. The time course for onset of symptoms with virilization is frequently reduced to months where symptoms relative to hirsutism may be present for years. This difference in time course and severity may be the result of tumor formation and, therefore, virilization must be evaluated rapidly and thoroughly.

THE ANDROGENS

Testosterone, androstenedione, and dehydroepiandrosterone (DHEA) are the major androgens produced and secreted into the circulation of the normal female. The quantity and activity of these androgens differs.

Testosterone is 5-10 times more potent than androstenedione and approximately 20 times more active than DHEA. Approximately 250 ug of testosterone are produced daily in the normal female. Of this, 50% is from glandular secretion divided equally between the adrenal glands and the ovaries. Of total testosterone production, 50% comes from the peripheral conversion of androstenedione. This conversion takes place via 17 ketosteroid reductase activity in the liver, muscle, skin, blood, and fat. Testosterone is mostly metabolized in the liver, however, some extraheptic conversion to dihydrotestosterone (DHT) takes place in the periphery. The metabolic clearance rate (MCR) for testosterone is approximately 650 liters per day.

Androstenedione is a weaker androgen but has a production rate 10 times that of testosterone. The average production rate for androstenedione is estimated to be 3 mg/day. Production of androstenedione is split with 50% ovarian production and 50% adrenal production. These relative contributions can vary due to adrenal circadian rhythm and an increased ovarian contribution at midcycle. Although the majority of androstenedione is metabolized in the liver, important peripheral conversion to testosterone and estrone does occur. The metabolic clearance rate of androstenedione is approximately 2000 liters per day.

Dehydroepiandosterone is the most abundant androgen secreted in the normal female. Its total production rate is probably greater than 10 mg/day. Approximately 90% of DHEA is derived from the adrenal glands providing an excellent marker for adrenal gland androgen production. The sulfated form of DHEA has a very low metabolic clearance rate (MCR) and, therefore, a long half-life. This provides a stable serum level and allows accurate evaluation with a single serum specimen.

Testosterone-Estradiol Binding Globulin (TEBG)

Androgens circulate in the blood bound to several plasma proteins. Sex steroid hormone binding globulin (SHBG) or testosterone estradiol binding globulin (TEBG) is a 30,000 molecular

weight liver generated β-globulin which has high affinity and a low
capacity for testosterone. Approximately 78% of the circulating
testosterone is bound to TEBG. However, 20% is bound to albumin in
a low affinity and high capacity situation. Approximately 1% of
testosterone circulates bound to transcortin. This leaves
approximately 1% of the circulating testosterone in a free unbound
form which is thought to be the biologically active portion of
testosterone. Anything that alters the quantity or function of TEBG
directly influences the amount of free testosterone available to
interact with tissues. Decreases in TEBG occur in liver and renal
disease and under the influence of increased total androgens. In
contrast, TEBG can be increased under the influence of estrogens and
thyroid hormones as well as during pregnancy. TEBG also binds
DHT and E_2. TEBG affinity for estradiol is about 75% relative to
testosterone, while affinity for DHT is twice that for testosterone.
Circulating androstenedione and DHEAS are bound only to albumin and
not to a specific binding globulin.

Most hirsute women have elevated production rates of
androstenedione and/or testosterone. Since androgens cause a
decrease TEBG binding capacity and an increase in the rate of
peripheral tissue extraction, excess androgens increase their own
MCR. This can produce normal or only slightly elevated serum levels
of testosterone and androstenedione in women who show increased
androgenic effect.

RAPID DIAGNOSTIC APPROACH TO HIRSUTISM

Establishing a precise diagnosis in patients with hirsutism is
important for two reasons:

Rule out serious disease (tumor, CAH).

Etiology of hyperandrogenism will dictate best therapy to
accomplish patients' therapeutic goals.

A rapid dignostic approach to hirsutism/hyperandrogenism should
include:

I. History

The important points to cover in the history include:
familial/ethnic background, other hirsute family members, age of
menarche, menstrual cyclicity, age of onset for hirsutism, time
course and severity of hirsutism, and drug history.

II. Physical Examination

Special attention should be directed toward a quantitation of the hirsute process. Evidence of virilism would include temporal balding, cliteromegaly, decrease in breast size, increase in muscle mass, and deepening of the voice. Clinical evidence of Cushing's syndrome should be sought. The pelvic examination should carefully evaluate ovarian size and formation of external genitalia.

III. Laboratory Screen

A. Anovulatory patients - LH, FSH, prolactin, testosterone, DHEAS

B. Ovulatory patients - Testosterone, free testosterone, TEBG, DHEAS

C. 17 Ketosteroids (17KS) - is a 24-hour urine test which measures DHEA and its metabolic products, etiolocholanolone and androsterone. Androsterone is also a metabolic product of androstenedione. This test does not measure testosterone which is not a 17KS and is not metabolized to a 17KS. 17KS evlevations occur in conditions where DHEA and/or androstenedione are elevated, i.e., adrenal tumors. However, the rare testosterone-only producing adrenal tumors will not elevate 17KS and an occasional ovarian tumor will produce enough androstenedione to place the 17KS in tumor range suggestive of adrenal etiology. DHEAS is such a definitive adrenal marker that its serum value in combination with a serum testosterone have almost eliminated the need for 17KS determinations. (Reproduced by permission R.L. Rosenfield, J Reprod Med 11:88, 1973).

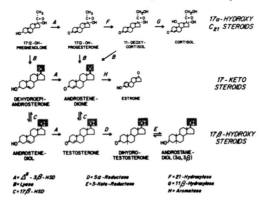

IV. <u>Other Testing to Rule Out</u>

   A. Adrenal Etiologies

      1. Cushing's syndrome - overnight dexamethasone
         suppression test, 24-hour urine free cortisol
      2. CAH - ACTH stimulation tests
      3. Tumor - ultrasound, CT scan, adrenal vein sampling.

   B. Ovarian Etiologies

      1. Tumor - ultrasound and surgery

ETIOLOGIES OF HIRSUTISM/HYPERANDROGENISM

   I. Idiopathic
  II. Ovarian
   A. Polycystic ovarian disease
   B. Hyperthecosis
   C. Tumor
 III. Adrenal
   A. Idiopathic
   B. Cushing's Sydrome
   C. Congenital Adrenal Hyperplasia
      1. 21-hydroxylase deficiency
      2. 11β-hydroxylase deficiency
      3. 3β-hydroxysteroid dehydrogenase deficiency
   D. Tumor
  IV. Medications

IDIOPATHIC HIRSUTISM

   Many patients presenting with hirsutism will not be found to
have any distinctive pathology. These patients may have genetic
predisposition which produces a hypersensitivity of certain hair
follicles to normal levels of circulating androgens. These patients
have normal menstrual cyclicity and no laboratory abnormalities can
be determined during their evaluation for hirsutism.

   There is some evidence that terminal hair growth is stimulated
by the 5α reduced form of testosterone, DHT. Increased production
of DHT secondary to increased 5α-reductase activity in the face of
otherwise normal testosterone levels could give rise to hirsutism
according to this theory. A major peripheral metabolite of DHT is
3-androstanediol-glucoronide. This substance has been found to be
elevated by several authors in cases of idiopathic hirsutism.

OVARIAN ETIOLOGIES

Clinical clues that may signify an ovarian etiology include:

1. Irregular menses, dysfunctional uterine bleeding
2. Obesity, hirsutism, acne
3. Family history positive for PCOD, hypertension, diabetes mellitus, endometrial carcinoma

A. <u>Polycystic ovarian disease</u> (PCOD) is the most common entity causing ovarian adrenal excess. PCOD is a classically described triad of obesity, oligomenorrhea, and hirsutism, however, there can be a wide spectrum of clinical presentation. PCOD occurs more frequently in certain families and is thought by some investigators to be inherited in an autosomal dominant pattern.

The pathophysiology of this disease is thought to relate to both hyperestrogenism and hyperandrogenism. Elevated androgens decrease TEBG and increase free estrogen and androgens. The estrogens provide a positive feedback on the pituitary to further increase LH production, and LH production further increases ovarian androgen production by the LH sensitive theca cells in the ovary. This milieu suppresses FSH production and cyclic ovulation does not occur. This "vicious-cycle" of PCOD can be exacerbated by obesity, stress, and exogenous androgenic hormones.

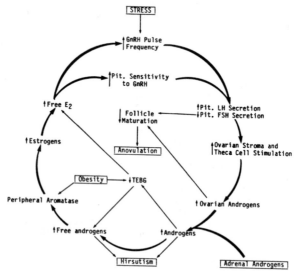

The laboratory findings in PCOD classically show:

1. An elevated serum LH to FSH ratio ($\geq$ 3:1)
2. Mildly elevated serum testosterone and androstenedione
3. A normal or slightly elevated serum DHEAS
4. A normal or slightly elevated serum prolactin

The onset of PCOD is classically at the time of menarche with a pattern of irregular menses thereafter. It should be noted that the cysts of the polycystic ovarian syndrome are very small, frequently measuring only 2-6 mm in size and the evaluation of ovarian size is the least helpful parameter for diagnosis and management of PCOD. Obesity is associated with increased levels of plasma testosterone and androstenedione and decreased amounts of TEBG. It can create or worsen the abnormal endocrine dynamics of PCOD. Weight loss will frequently reverse the above and should be strongly encouraged.

B. Hyperthecosis may be an exaggerated form of PCOD. However, the ovarian defect seems to be in the ovarian stroma rather than related to multiple follicle cysts. The presentation of hyperthecosis is similar to PCOD, however, the hyperandrogenism is generally worse and often leads to virilization.

The laboratory findings frequently show:
1. A normal LH value
2. A LH/FSH ratio < 2
3. Serum testosterone value 100-200 ng/dl.

These findings give a presentation similar to ovarian tumors.

C. Ovarian tumors can produce hirsutism and hyperandrogenism. Suspect an ovarian tumor if:

1. Serum testosterone is > 200 ng/dl
2. Serum testosterone value is > 2.5 times the upper limit of normal for any assay
3. Normal DHEAS
4. Rapid onset of hirsutism (6-12 months)
5. Evidence of virilization

Ovarian tumors associated with increased androgens include lipoid cell tumors, leydig cell tumors, arrhenoblastomas, dysgerminomas, brenner cell tumors, teratomas, cystadenomas, cystadenocarcinomas, luteomas, and hyperreactio luteinalis. Although some of these tumors can achieve a large dimension, others are very small making diagnosis sometimes difficult. Initial evaluation should include a good bimanual pelvic examination and pelvic ultrasonography. If a tumor cannot be demonstrated, exploratory laparotomy must be performed to evaluate both ovaries surgically .

ADRENAL ETIOLOGIES

A. Idiopathic is the most common adrenal etiology for hirsutism. This form of hirsutism presents with mildly elevated DHEAS, elevated or normal testosterone, and slightly elevated urinary 17-ketosteroids. This diagnosis is one of exclusion after determining there is no evidence of Cushing's syndrome, congenital adrenal hyperplasia, or tumor.

B. Cushing's syndrome, excess production of glucocorticoids can present with hirsutism and irregular menses. However, the usual findings of centripetal obesity, abdominal striae, muscle wasting, hypertension, osteoporosis, and easy bruising often help make this diagnosis. Cushing's syndrome is diagnosed using the overnight dexamethasone suppression test.

Overnight Dexamethasone Suppression Test

Dexamethasone 1 mg orally at 11:00 PM
Serum Cortisol next morning at 8:00 AM

Serum Cortisol Value	Interpretation	Action
< 5 µg/dl	No Cushing's	None
> 5 µg/dl, < 10 ug/dl	Possible Cushing's	24-hour urine free cortisol test
> 10 µg/dl	Probable Cushing's	Refer for further testing/management

If the urine for free cortisol shows adequate creatinine for a 24-hour collection and greater than 90 µg/24-hour free cortisol, the patient should be referred for management of Cushing's syndrome.

C. The classic enzyme defects causing congenital adrenal hyperplasia (CAH) all have a nonclassical late onset form which presents after menarche with hirsutism and irregular menses. The enzyme defects are incomplete and may represent a heterozygote carrier state, an allelic variation of the classic defect, or both. These syndromes, like their more classic counterparts, are inherited as autosomal recessive traits.

The gene which codes for the 21-hydroxylase enzyme-cytochrome P450 complex has been sequenced and is located on the short arm of chromosome 6. Due to close proximity to the HLA region of this same chromosome, genetic linkage disequilibrium has been established between the HLA-Bw47 and DR7 loci and the classical 21OH deficiency genes as well as beween the HLA-B14 and DR1 loci and the late onset nonclassical 21OH deficiency genes. Unfortunately, the locations of the genes for 3β-hydroxysteroid dehydrogenase and 11β-hydroxylase are not known and linkage studies with HLA are not helpful in these diagnoses. Recently the gene for 11β-hydroxylase has been sequenced, however, and genetic probes may soon help in this diagnosis.

The 21-hydroxylase (21-OH) form of late onset CAH is by far the most common. The gene frequency of this disease varies in different patient populations from 1/27 among some Ashkenazi Jews to less than 1/1000 among Anglo-Saxons. This may explain the difference in prevalence among hirsute patients which has been reported as low as 1.2% and as high as 20% by different authors. As this gene has been sequenced and genetic probes are available, accurate diagnosis may soon be performed by DNA studies. However, at present, the laboratory diagnosis of this entity is made using an ACTH stimulation test. The baseline 17-hydroxyprogesterone values for individuals with a late onset 21-hydroxylase CAH are generally within normal range. Similarly, DHEAS and androstenedione may also be within the normal range.

ACTH Stimulation Test

1. Perform the test during the follicular phase of the menstrual cycle in ovulatory women.
2. Draw baseline serum progesterone (P_0) and 17-OH progesterone (17-OH P_0).
3. Administer 1 mg (4 ampules of 0.25 mg) cortrosyn intravenously.
4. After 30 minutes, draw another serum progesterone (P_{30}) and 17-OH progesterone (17-OH P_{30}).
5. Convert all serum values to ng/dl.
6. Calculate a combined rate of increase using the following formula:

$$\frac{(P_{30} - P_0) + (17\text{-OH } P_{30} - 17\text{-OH } P_0)}{30 \text{ minutes}}$$

7. A value of greater than 6.8 ng/dl/minute is indicative of partial 21-hydroxylase deficiency.

A late onset partial 3β-hydroxysteroid dehydrogenase deficiency has been described among hirsute women. The criteria for diagnosis, however, are not well standardized. Baseline 17-OH pregnenolone and

DHEAS are elevated in most cases. The 17-OH pregnenolone to 17-hydroxyprogesterone ratio may be elevated before (greater than 4 to 1) and after stimulation with synthetic ACTH 0.25 mg IV (greater than 6 to 1).

A late onset partial defect of 11β-hydroxylase has also been defined among hirsute women. However, the criteria for making this diagnosis are again not standardized. Baseline elevations in serum 11-desoxycortisol (compound S) and its major urinary metabolite, tetrahydro-11-desoxycortisol may exist, and these compounds are elevated after ACTH stimulation. However, the exact values will depend upon individual laboratories.

D. Tumors

Neoplasms of the adrenal glands, adenomas or carcinomas, frequently cause signs of Cushing's syndrome, however, they may present with simple virilization.

Suspect an adrenal tumor if:

1. Serum testosterone is > 200 ng/dl and/or serum DHEAS is > 700 ug/dl.
2. Serum values for testosterone and/or DHEAS are greater than 2.5 times the upper limit of normal in any assay.
3. Urinary 17-ketosteroids are > 50 g/24 hours.
4. Rapid onset of hirsutism (6-12 months).
5. Evidence of virilization.

Several cases of pure testosterone producing adenomas have been reported. As testosterone is not measured in the 17-ketosteroid assay, these particular cases would not be picked up by screening with 17-ketosteroids alone. Once a tentative diagnosis of adrenal tumor is made on the basis of screening tests, definitive imaging with either ultrasound or CT scan should be performed. Fortunately, most adrenal neoplasms are greater than 1 cm in diameter which allows accurate detection by CT or ultrasound scanning. In difficult or equivocal cases, selective adrenal vein sampling can be performed. Invasive venography can be dangerous, has been reported to give confusing results, and should only be used as a last resort. Gonadotropin responsive adrenal tumors, ACTH responsive ovarian tumors, and suggestions that dexamethasone may be capable of inhibiting ovarian androgen biosynthesis significantly limit the benefit of stimulation-suppression testing in differentiating adrenal from ovarian tumors.

MEDICATIONS

Hirsutism can be drug-induced by a number of medications including:

1. Anabolic steroids - used by "body-builders"
2. Danazol - used for the treatment of endometriosis
3. 19-nor progestins - used for progestational effects
4. Dilantin - used to prevent grand mal seizures

THERAPY

I. Identify and surgically remove ovarian/adrenal tumor
II. Identify and treat Cushing's syndrome or CAH
III. Treatment for patients not desiring pregnancy
  A. Suppress Ovarian Function
    1. Combination oral contraceptives
    2. Medroxyprogesterone acetate
  B. Suppress Adrenal Function
    1. Dexamethasone
    2. Prednisone
  C. Antiandrogen Therapy
    1. Spironolactone
    2. Cimetidine
    3. Cyproterone acetate
IV. Treatment for patients desiring pregnancy
  A. Ovulation Induction
    1. Clomid
    2. Human menopausal gonadotropins
    3. Pure FSH
    4. Dexamethasone
V. No Treatment

Therapy must be individualized for each patient. The etiology of the hirsutism/hyperandrogenism must be found and treated appropriately. Ovarian and adrenal tumors must be identified and surgically removed. Similarly, Cushing's syndrome needs to be identified and referred for appropriate therapy. The other etiologies for hirsutism require medications that provide either ovarian suppression, adrenal suppression, or antiandrogen effects by binding to the androgen receptor.

Ovarian suppression is accomplished with the use of combination oral contraceptives. These provide multiple benefits to the hirsute patient including an increase in TEBG causing a decrease in free steroid hormones; a reduction in serum LH causing a decrease in ovarian androgen output; a decrease in serum DHEAS reflecting some effect on the adrenal gland; cyclic menstrual flow avoiding development of endometrial hyperplasia; and provide contraception. This combination of benefits makes use of oral contraceptives the primary choice for the treatment of hirsutism in the patient not desiring pregnancy. Individuals unable to take oral contraceptives secondary to contraindications may benefit from the use of the medroxyprogesterone acetate, 30 mg a day. This regimen will decrease LH and ovarian androgen output and protect the endometrium from hyperplasia. However, it has little effect on the adrenal gland and does not elevate TEBG.

Adrenal suppression is accomplished with the use of dexamethasone, 0.25-0.75 mg orally at bedtime. Dexamethasone will decrease the ACTH-dependent androgen synthesis in the adrenal gland and may have a limited effect on ovarian androgen production. Although dexamethasone will suppress glucocorticoids in 24 hours, it takes approximately 6-8 weeks for a similar suppression of adrenal androgens. Patients on long term suppressive therapy should be monitored with an 8 AM cortisol. This value should be equal to or greater than 3 ug/dl to ensure there is not suppression of the pituitary adrenal axis.

Antiandrogens are especially recommended for the treatment of hirsutism associated with increased end organ sensitivity. These compounds selectively inhibit the binding of DHT to its receptor, thereby blocking the androgenic effect. All of these compounds have the potential through this mechanism to feminize the external genitalia of a male fetus when administered to a pregnant mother. Therefore, careful attention must be directed to contraception for these patients. Often these medications can be combined with dexamethasone or oral contraceptives for a combined approach to the treatment of hirsutism. Cyproterone acetate has been extensively used in European countries, however, it is not approved for use in the United States. Cimetidine is a histamine receptor antagonist as well as an androgen receptor antagonist. Its use in the treatment of hirsutism requires up to 1500 mg/day. Side-effects at that dose can include diarrhea, dizziness, muscle pain, and leukopenia. Spironolactone is a aldosterone antagonist and antiandrogen which was originally developed as an antihypertensive agent. It appears to increase the MCR of testosterone and decreases the synthesis rate of testosterone as well as its effects at the level of the receptor. This medication is given in doses of 50-200 mg/day orally. At this dose, side-effects sometimes include headache, nausea, weakness, and lassitude. These effects are not secondary to elevated serum potassium and seemed to improve after several months of therapy.

In conjunction with the medical therapies or in place of them, various cosmetic treatments can be undertaken. These include bleaching, shaving, depilatory creams, plucking, waxing, and electrolysis. Only electrolysis is a permanent form of hair removal, the others needing repetition at various intervals.

Hirsute patients are frequently anovulatory and desirous of pregnancy. These patients are treated with ovulation induction utilizing clomiphene citrate, hMG, or most recently, pure FSH (see Chapter 11). Only in patients with severe resistance to regimens of ovulation induction should an ovarian wedge resection be considered. Severe adhesion formation can cause iatrogenic infertility in patients undergoing ovarian wedge resections. Microsurgical technique with the use of fine suture (5-0, 6-0) should be used for ovarian repair. Patients desiring pregnancy should not receive antiandrogen therapy.

Patients may elect no therapy. These patients should be reminded of the risk chronic oligo- or anovulation carries for causing intermittent episodes of dysfunctional bleeding and potential endometrial hyperplasia. An anovulatory patient should be encouraged to use a cyclic progestin to prevent endometrial hyperplasia. Medroxyprogesterone acetate, 10 mg a day for 10-14 days each month is adequate. Patients should also be counseled that they may ovulate intermittently, and if they do not desire pregnancy they should use some form of contraception.

When treating hirsute patients remember:

1. Therapy must be continuous for 6-9 months before significant results can be expected.
2. A combination of medical therapies may be more beneficial than single therapy.
3. Frequently medical therapy must be combined with hair removal to achieve an adequate result.
4. Although increased androgens are needed to stimulate the transformation of vellus to terminal hair, terminal hair growth may continue at normal androgen levels.
5. The rate of hair growth increases during summer months.

SUGGESTED READING

Abraham GE: Ovarian and adrenal contribution to peripheral androgens during the menstrual cycle. J Clin Endocrinol Metabol 39:340, 1974.

Gabrilove JL, Seman AT, Sabet R, Mitty HA, Nicolis GL: Virilizing adrenal adenoma with studies on the steroid content of the adrenal

venus effluent and a review of the literature. Endocrinol Rev
2:462, 1981.

Horton R, Hawks D, Lobo R: 3, 17-androstanediol gludoronide in
plasma, a marker of androgen action in idiopathic hirsutism. J Clin
Invest 69:1203, 1982.

Lobo RA, Paul WL, Goebelsmann U: Dehydroepiandrosterone sulfate as
an indicator of adrenal androgen function. Obstet Gynecol 57:69,
1981.

Maroulis GB: Evaluation of hirsutism and hyperandrogenemia. Fertil
Steril 36:273, 1981.

Mauvais-Jarvis P, Kuttenn F, Mowszowicz I: Hirsutism. Monographs
on Endocrinology. Springer-Verlag, New York, 1981.

Pittaway DE, Maxson WS, Wentz AC: Spironolactone in combination
drug therapy for unresponsive hirsutism. Fertil Steril 43:878,
1985.

Wiebe RH (Ed): Androgenology in Women. Seminars in Reproductive
Endocrinology Vol 4 No. 2, 1986.

Yen SSC: The polycystic ovary syndrome. Clin Endocrinol 12:177,
1980.

Chapter 7

The Thyroid and Its Disorders

George A. Hill, M.D.

THYROID FUNCTION

INTRODUCTION

Thyroid homeostasis is modulated by a complex set of interrelated mechanisms. Thyrotropin releasing hormone (TRH), synthesized by the anterior hypothalamus is transported to the anterior pituitary via the hypothalamic pituitary portal system. This stimulates secretion of thyroid stimulating hormone (TSH) by the anterior pituitary which directly stimulates the thyroid gland. There are also numerous autoregulatory mechanisms within the thyroid gland itself.

The biologically active thyroid hormones include thyroxine (T_4) and triiodothyronine (T_3). Although T_4 is secreted at 8-10 times the rate of T_3, T_3 is 3-4 times more potent. T_3 is the active thyroid hormone. Within the thyroid gland cell nucleus, the thyroid hormone receptor has a 10-fold higher affinity for T_3 over T_4. T_4 metabolism is also in the direction of T_3. About 30% of T_4 produced daily is converted by monodeiodination to T_3 and about 40% is converted to reverse T_3 (rT_3) which has little if any biologic effect. T_3 measurements are an indirect reflection of thyroid function, with about 80% being derived from T_4; starvation, stress and other factors inhibit the conversion. Although these hormones feedback at the level of the pituitary to influence TSH secretion, the relationship between TSH, T_4, and T_3 is complex and not totally understood.

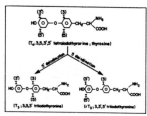

Structures of T_4, T_3, and rT_3

Hormones Involved in Thyroid Function

Serum Thyroxine (T4): Serum T_4 levels by radioimmunoassay (RIA) are affected by thyroidal secretion of T_4 and the serum binding capacity for T_4. Over 99% of the T_4 circulating is bound to the serum proteins thyroxine binding globulin (TBG), thyroxine binding prealbumin (TBPA), and albumin. To interpret the level of T_4, one needs to know the serum T_4 binding capacity. The daily production of T_4 is about 90 µg, and the half-life is 8 days.

Free Thyroxine (FT4): Free T_4 (unbound) is the metabolically active hormone fraction. It accounts for less than 0.1% of the total T_4 circulating in the blood and has little or no direct effect on tissues. T_4 serves mainly as a precursor for T_3. The assay for free T_4 is a technically difficult test to perform.

Thyroid Binding Globulin (TBG): The level of TBG affects the level of T_4 as well as T_3. Numerous factors may affect TBG levels:

INCREASED TBG	DECREASED TBG
Estrogen therapy	Androgen therapy
Pregnancy	Severe hypoproteinemia
Acute hepatitis	Chronic liver disease
Acute intermittent porphyria	Glucocorticoid excess
Hereditary TBG increase	Hereditary TBG deficiency
Neonatal state	Acromegaly
Biliary cirrhosis	

T3 Resin Uptake (T3rU): The T_3rU measures indirectly the number of unoccupied protein binding sites for T_4 and T_3 in serum. Radiolabeled T_3 is added to the patient's serum and competes for binding sites on the TBG molecule. Radiolabeled T_3 is used instead of T_4 because the assay time is shorter. An inert material is then added to absorb any unbound radiolabeled T_3. The radioactivity of the resin is counted and expressed as percent of total counts added to the assay tube. It is important to note that this test measures

T_4 and not T_3. In all cases, the T_3rU is inversely proportional to the number of available binding sites on TBG.

Hyperthyroidism	↑T_4	↓ Availability of binding sites on TBG	↓ Binding of labeled T_3 on TBG	↑T_3rU
Hypothyroidism	↓T_4	↑ Availability of binding sites on TBG	↑ Binding of labeled T_3 on TBG	↓T_3rU
Hypoproteinemia	nl T_4	↓ Availability of binding sites on TBG	↓ Binding of labeled T_3 on TBG	↑T_3rU
Hyperproteinemia	nl T_4	↑ Availability of binding sites on TBG	↑ Binding of labeled T_3 on TBG	↓T_3rU

Free Thyroxine Index (FTI): This gives an estimate of the unbound or free T_4 and is calculated as shown below.

$$FTI = \text{Total } T_4 \times \frac{\text{Patients } T_3rU}{\text{Mean normal } T_3rU}$$

3, 5, 3' Triiodothyronine (T_3): T_3 is the metabolically active thyroid hormone which binds to nuclear receptors of target tissues, and is found when T_4 is deiodinated into T_3. T_3 circulates in the blood at concentrations 50 times lower than T_4. T_3 circulates largely bound to proteins and the free fraction (0.1%) is responsible for its effects. Serum T_3 (RIA) is useful in iodine deficient states where the T_4 may be low. Approximately 30 µg of T_3 are produced daily, the majority outside the thyroid from circulating T_4. The half-life of T_3 is 16 hours.

Thyroid Stimulating Hormone-Thyrotropin (TSH): TSH is a glycoprotein secreted by the pituitary gland and regulated by a classical negative feedback system dependent on the level of FT_4. TSH is a glycoprotein of molecular weight 28000 Daltons consisting of 2 noncovalently linked subunits α and β. The uniqueness of TSH is determined by its β subunit, since the α subunit is identical to the α subunit in FSH and LH. TSH stimulates thyroid growth as well as synthesis and secretion of thyroid hormones. Both T_4 and T_3 inhibit TSH output, but evidence suggests that intrapituitary deiodination of T_4 to T_3 is important in regulation. Serum TSH is measured by RIA and is essential in diagnosing primary hypothyroidism.

TRH: TRH is a tripeptide secreted by the hypothalamus which
circulates to the pituitary via the hypophyseal portal system. TRH
stimulates thyrotropes in the pituitary to secrete TSH. TRH
administration is useful in states where hyperthyroidism is
suspected and the diagnosis is not clear using static determinations.
The TRH test is performed as follows:

1. A baseline TSH is drawn at time 0.
2. TRH (500 μg) is given IV over 15-20 seconds.
3. Blood is drawn for TSH determination at 30 minutes.

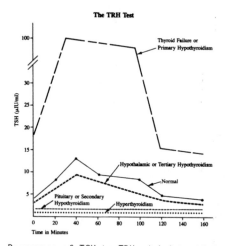

Responses of TSH to TRH administration

Thyroidal 24-Hour Radioactive Iodine Uptake (RAIU): The
thyroid gland concentrates iodine which it uses for thyroxine
synthesis, so measurement of the uptake of radioactive iodine is a
useful marker of thyroid function. The RAIU is calculated as the
percentage of total administered radioactivity taken up by the
thyroid and this is usually made 24 hours after an oral ingestion of
tracer doses of ^{131}I (or ^{123}I). This test is rarely used as a
primary diagnostic aid.

If the thyroid gland is not functioning, then the 24-hour RAIU
is low. If the iodine content of the plasma pool is elevated

secondary to the ingestion of iodine rich foods, medications, or radiographic agents, the 24-hour value for tracer uptake may be low even though thyroid function is normal. In a diffuse toxic goiter the thyroidal trapping of iodine is increased and the 24-hour ^{131}I uptake will be elevated. All radionuclide tests are contraindicated during pregnancy.

Thyroid Imaging or Scan: Radionuclide imaging of the thyroid is useful in ascertaining whether or not an area of the thyroid is functioning. The most often used radiotracers are technetium-99M pertechnetate, ^{131}I, and ^{125}I.

Recovery of Thyroid Function After Prolonged Suppression

Patients with endocrine and infertility problems are often found to be taking thyroid hormone without evidence of hypothyroidism. After the abrupt withdrawal of chronic suppressive thyroid hormone therapy from intrinsically euthyroid persons, a period of decreased pituitary thyrotropin reserve ensues, and patients generally complain of fatigue. Return of the serum T_4 concentrations into the normal range requires at least 3 weeks, and sometimes up to 6 weeks. The return of ^{131}I uptake into the normal range usually requires only 2-4 weeks and generally coincides with the return of detectable concentrations of TSH in the serum. Therefore, thyroid function should be measured at least 6 weeks after discontinuation of replacement thyroid hormone.

HYPERTHYROIDISM

Hyperthyroidism is the syndrome which develops after body tissues are exposed to increased concentrations of T_4 and/or T_3. T_3 may be elevated to a greater degree than T_4. TSH is usually undetectable.

In the elderly the classical signs are often not present and hyperthyroidism may present with dysrhythmias or heart failure as well as weight loss, weakness, or anorexia.

The most sensitive test for hyperthyroidism is the TRH test. Absence of the normal rise in TSH secretion indicates suppression of the hypothalamic pituitary axis and, thus, the likelihood of hyperthyroidism. A normal response of TSH to TRH virtually excludes the diagnosis of hyperthyroidism.

SYMPTOMS	SIGNS
Nervousness	Thyroid enlargement
Increased perspiration	Tremor
Heat intolerance	Hyperkinesis
Palpitations	Exophthalmos
Weight loss	Lid retraction
Dyspnea	Lid lag
Fatigue	Tachycardia
Weakness	Smooth and velvety skin
Increased appetite	Moist and warm hands
Hyperdefecation	Onycholysis (plummer's nails)
Menstrual dysfunction	Thyroid bruit
Eye symptoms	
Swelling of legs	
Diarrhea	

Graves Disease

Graves disease is the most common cause of hyperthyroidism and is 8 times more common in females than males. It is distinguished clinically from other forms of hyperthyroidism by the presence of diffuse thyroid enlargement, ophthalmopathy, and occasionally pretibal myxedema. Graves disease is an immunological disorder in which thyroid stimulating immunoglobulins bind to the TSH receptors on follicular cells causing thyroidogenesis.

CAUSES OF HYPERTHYROIDISM

Subacute thyroiditis	Toxic multinodular goiter
Painless thyroiditis	Toxic adenoma
Exogenous hyperthyroidism	TSH-producing tumor
Factituous hyperthyroidism	Iodine-induced hyperthyroidism
Iatrogenic hyperthyroidism	Thyroid storm

Treatment of Hyperthyroidism: Treatment involves controlling the hyperthyroidism with antithyroid drugs until the basic disease process undergoes spontaneous remission. Since spontaneous remission only occurs in approximately 20-30% of patients in the United States, the clinician must decide on long-term antithyroid medication or some form of ablative thyroid therapy.

1. Antithyroid Drugs: Thionamides, propylthiouracil (PTU) and methimazole (Tapazole), block thyroid peroxidase and, thus, inhibit thyroid hormone biosynthesis by blocking iodide organification, and block the coupling reaction. Both drugs have weak immunosuppressive effects and PTU has an

inhibitory effect on the conversion of T_4 to T_3. PTU is bound extensively to serum albumin, while methimazole is not bound appreciably to serum proteins. Antithyroid drugs are actively concentrated by the thyroid gland. Treatment consists of PTU, 100-300 mg TID, or methimazole, 10-30 mg TID, until the serum T_3 by RIA is normal. Complications of thionamides include fever, rash, urticaria, arthralgia, arthritis, and agranulocytosis. Leukopenia is the most common side-effect. Routine blood counts are not predictive of this toxic effect. The patient must be told to come immediately for a complete blood count if there is fever, sore throat, or diarrhea. Fever, myalgias, and lupus-like syndromes may also occur but generally remit when the drug is discontinued.

PHARMACOLOGICAL FEATURES OF ANTITHYROID DRUGS

	PTU	Methimazole
Serum protein binding	High	Low
Serum half-life	75 minutes	4-6 hours
Transplacental passage	Low	High
Levels in breast milk	Low	High
Teratogenesis		Cutis aplasia

2. Radioactive Iodine Therapy: ^{131}I therapy is the treatment of choice for most adults with Graves disease. Within 6-12 weeks after ^{131}I, the patient is generally euthyroid. If the patient is still hyperthyroid 6-12 months after ^{131}I, a second treatment is necessary. Hypothyroidism develops in approximately 20-70% of patients. Patients treated with ^{131}I must be continuously monitored for evidence of hypothyroidism.

3. Surgery: Subtotal thyroidectomy is infrequently used in the treatment of hyperthyroidism.

4. β-Adrenergic Antagonist: Propranolol is the most commonly used β blocker and alleviates many of the symptoms of hyperthyroidism. The usual dose is 20-40 mg QID. Propranolol is especially useful in the treatment of thyroid crisis.

5. Iodine: Inorganic iodine inhibits thyroid hormone synthesis and release. Five to ten drops of saturated solution of potassium iodine TID will reduce the serum T_4 and T_3 by 50% within 7-14 days. Then T_4 and T_3 return to previous levels in most patients.

THYROID STORM

Thyroid storm accounts for much of the mortality associated with hyperthyroidism. Thyroid storm is characterized as a state of unregulated hypermetabolism with fever and tachycardia and almost always occurs in patients with pre-existant hyperthyroidism due to diffuse toxic goiter. These patients have excess sympathetic (adrenergic) activity and show markedly increased effects of thyroid hormone.

SIGNS AND SYMPTOMS OF THYROID STORM

Signs

Endocrine
  Thyromegaly
  Exophthalmus
Systemic
  Hyperpyrexia
  Sweating
Cardiovascular
  Tachycardia, arrhythmias
  Congestive heart failure
Gastrointestinal
  Hepatomegaly
Nervous system
  Hyperreflexia
  Tremor
  Coma
  Irritability

Symptoms

Cardiovascular
  Palpitations
  Dyspena
  Edema
Gastrointestinal
  Vomiting
  Diarrhea
  Jaundice
  Weight loss
Nervous system
  Weakness
  Apathy
  Psychosis

CRITERIA FOR THYROID STORM

1. Temperature greater than 100°F
2. Marked tachycardia out of proportion to the fever
3. Exaggerated manifestations of thyrotoxicosis
4. Dysfunction of the central nervous system, cardiovascular system, or gastrointestinal system

Thyroid storm is generally precipitated by a medical or surgical insult, for example, infection, toxemia of pregnancy, or surgery. The diagnosis is based on a careful clinical history and physical examination. There are no specific laboratory tests to indicate the presence of thyroid storm. The serum concentrations of T_3 or T_4 will not differentiate patients with thyroid storm from patients with hyperthyroidism.

Treatment is directed at decreasing both the synthesis and release of thyroid hormones, as well as blocking the increased adrenergic activity. For thyroid storm, PTU should be administered in amounts of 900-1200 mg/day. A decline in T_3 levels requires 24 hours of therapy, and a decrease in the level of T_4 takes 4-6 days. Iodine administration will inhibit the release of T_3 and T_4 from the thyroid within a few hours. β-Blockade (propranolol) rapidly reverses the adrenergic effects seen in thyroid storm,however, these drugs are contraindicated in patients with chronic lung disease or in patients with heart block. Plasmapheresis to remove large amounts of protein bound thyroid hormone may be needed in patients who do not respond to other measures.

HYPOTHYROIDISM

Hypothyroidism develops when there is an inadequate affect of thyroid hormone on body tissues. Over 99% of cases are caused by deficient production of thyroid hormones by the thyroid gland leading to low serum levels of T_4. In hypothyroidism, the tissues are infiltrated by hydrophilic mucopolysaccharides leading to the nonpitting edema termed myxedema.

TYPES OF HYPOTHYROIDISM

	Serum T_4	Serum TSH	TSH RESPONSE
1^0 (Thyroid)	↓	↑	↑
2^0 (Pituitary)	↓	↓	Absent
3^0 (Hypothalamus)	↓	↓	Normal

Severe hypothyroidism can lead to coma and respiratory compromise. Congenital hypothyroidism is associated with mental retardation. Juvenile hypothyroidism is characterized by epiphyseal dysgenesis and short stature.

92

SYMPTOMS	SIGNS
Marked cold intolerance	Rough, scaly, dry, cool skin
Weakness	Pallid or yellow tinted skin
Muscle cramps	Nonpitting edema of the eyelids, hands, and feet
Aching	Slow movements
Stiffness	Slowness of thought
Hoarseness	Slow relaxation time of deep tendon reflexes
Decreased hearing	Bradycardia
Paresthesias	Cardiac failure
Mild weight gain despite a normal appetite	Pericardial effusion
Constipation and ileus	Hypertension
Dry skin	
Decreased perspiration	
Somnolence	

Causes of Hypothyroidism

1. Primary hypofunction
   A. Insufficient amount of functional thyroid tissue
      Primary atrophy of the thyroid gland
      Chronic thyroiditis
      Prior ^{131}I treatment
      Prior thyroid surgery
      Thyroid agenesis
   B. Defective biosynthesis of thyroid hormone
      Iodine deficiency
      Congenital defects of trapping
      Congenital defects of organification of iodine
      Excessive antithyroid medications
      Iodine excess

2. Secondary Hypothyroidism

   A. Related to pituitary diseases
      Pituitary tumor

Diagnosis

Hypothyroidism is confirmed by finding a low serum T_4 and T_3rU. Antibodies to thyroid microsomes or thyroglobulin are usually present in autoimmune thyroid disease. Anemia is often present. Serum cholesterol and triglycerides may be elevated. Serum T_3 (RIA) is generally not helpful because over one-half of patients with hypothyroidism have levels within the normal range.

Nongoitrous Hypothyroidism

Spontaneous primary thyroid atrophy: No goiter is present.
The female to male ratio is 6 to 1. There is a loss of tissue as a
result of destruction leading to fibrosis and atrophy. This may be
associated with failure of other endocrine organs.

Goitrous Hypothyroidism

Chronic autoimmune thyroiditis (Hashimoto's thyroiditis): This
is the most common disease of the thyroid gland. Diffuse
enlargement of the thyroid gland is associated with high titers of
thyroid autoantibodies. Histologically the thyroid has large
amounts of lymphocyte infiltration with follicular hypertrophy.

Drug-induced hypothyroidism
Hypothyroidism due to iodine deficiency
Dyshormonogenesis
Postablative hypothyroidism

Euthyroid sick: Patients with nonthyroidal illnesses may have
abnormal thyroid tests:
1. Low T_4 with normal FT_4
2. Low or high FT_4
3. Low T_3 and FT_3
4. Slightly elevated TSH with normal or increased
   response to TRH
5. Decreased TSH with blunted response to TRH

Treatment of Hypothyroidism

Thyroid Replacement: L-thyroxine is prescribed in a dose of 2
µg/kg body weight per day with the average replacement dose being
approximately 150-200 µg/day. Advantages of its use include:
1. Assured potency
2. Single daily dose
3. Inexpensive
4. Constant levels of serum T_4
5. The ability to assess adequacy of replacement by
   measuring serum T_4 (RIA).

In the young, mildly hypothyroid patient one may start with
the full replacement dose of L-thyroxine. However, for the severely
hypothyroid patient, gradual replacement is indicated in order to
avoid cardiovascular problems. In these patients, L-thyroxine,
0.025 mg/day, is prescribed for 2-3 three weeks and then increased
by 0.025 mg/day every 2-3 weeks until maintenance dose is reached.

T_3 is not routinely used in the treatment of hypothyroidism for the following reasons:
1) Peaks of T_3 following absorption in the GI tract are much higher than normal
2) T_3 must be taken TID
3) It is considerable more expensive
4) Serum T_4 cannot be used to assess replacement therapy

Simple Nontoxic Goiter

In simple nontoxic goiter, found often in young women who present with enlargement of the anterior neck, the thyroid may be just palpable or moderately enlarged. However, it is generally soft and nontender without palpable nodules. The patient is asymptomatic and chemically euthyroid. No evidence of thyroid autoantibodies can be found or they are present in low titers. This patient may be followed to see if the thyroid will continue to enlarge or may be begun on thyroid suppression if the gland is moderately enlarged.

THYROID NODULES

Thyroid nodules may be found in up to 5% of the female population. The biggest concern in patients with thyroid nodules is establishing whether the nodule is benign or malignant. Risk factors for thyroid carcinoma include:

1. Age: One-half of thyroid nodules in children less than 16 years old are malignant, therefore, they should be excised.
2. Sex: Thyroid nodules are 5 times more common in females than males, however, thyroid carcinoma is only 2 times more common in females than males; therefore, a thyroid nodule in a male has a higher chance of being malignant than in a female.
3. History of irradiation: Irradiation of the head and neck is associated with an increased risk of thyroid carcinoma, therefore, patients with a nodule and this history should have the nodule excised.
4. History of familial thyroid carcinoma
5. Physical characteristics of the thyroid gland:

Benign	Malignant
Multinodular	Single nodule
"Hot" hyperfunctioning	Rapidly enlarging
nodules	Firm, irregular nodule
Simple cyst	Adherent to overlying
	muscle
	"Cold" on scan

Work Up and Management of the Thyroid Nodule

1. History and physical examination: Look for enlarged lymph nodes in the neck and the physical characteristics of the gland.
2. Draw serum T_4 (RIA), T_3rU, thyroid antimicrosomal antibodies.
3. Obtain thyroid scintiscan to see if the nodule is functioning.
4. If there is any suspicion of malignancy, surgical excision is recommended.
5. If there is no suspicion of malignancy, fine needle aspiration is performed.
6. Thyroid suppressive therapy: Since most nodules are responsive to TSH, try treating with L-thyroxine. One can suppress the TSH and maintain the euthyroid status with this treatment.
   a. Thyroid suppression is continued for 3-6 months.
   b. If the nodule decreases > 50%, continue suppressive therapy.
   c. If the nodule decreases < 50%, re-evaluation is indicted.
   d. If a nodule grows during suppressive therapy, surgical excision is mandatory.

THYROID CHANGES DURING PREGNANCY

Mild forms of hypothyroidism or hyperthyroidism do not alter chances of conception. In severe forms of hypothyroidism, however, low levels of serum T_4 result in increased TRH. With increased TRH, secretion of prolactin as well as TSH is stimulated. Prolactin may inhibit the LH surge at the level of GnRH and result in anovulation. Hyperthyroidism generally does not affect the rate of conception, however, it may result in an increased incidence of fetal wastage and stillbirths. During pregnancy, the thyroid enlarges and takes up more iodine, the basal metabolic rate increases, and levels of total T_4 rise. However, there is no increase in thyroid hormone secretion.

Change in Laboratory Values: The rise in estrogen associated with pregnancy promotes the synthesis of thyroid-binding globulin

(TBG) by the liver. As a result, the levels of total T_4 in plasma
rise. However, FT_4 and FT_3 levels remain unchanged. Therefore, in
pregnancy thyroid function should be assessed by measurement of free
T_4.

Management of Thyroid Disease During Pregnancy: The increase
in steroid hormone production during pregnancy suppresses the
formation of IgG and IgA antibodies. This may result in improvement
of pre-existing hyperthyroidism or hypothyroidism due to Graves
disease or Hashimoto's thyroiditis during pregnancy. However, a
rebound phenomenon may occur postpartum.

Hypothyroidism should be recognized before pregnancy and
treated with replacement therapy. Patients with hyperthyroidism
should be initially treated with antithyroid drugs such as
Propylthiouracil 100 mg TID and then reduce the dose subsequently if
possible, since these drugs cross the placenta and may inhibit the
fetal thyroid gland. A mild degree of hyperthyroidism during
pregnancy is usually well tolerated.

THYROID CHANGES IN THE NEONATE

Maternal TSH and T_4 do not cross the placental barrier. The
fetus' regulation of thyroid function is under its own pituitary
control which is fully active during the last trimester of pregnancy.
Prior to birth, T_4 levels are normal and there is a relative
deficiency of T_3 and excessive levels of rT_3 presumably due to
abnormal peripheral deiodination of T_4. Within 30 minutes of birth,
TSH levels rise and peak. This rise in TSH promotes increases in
both T_4 and T_3. T_3 peaks at 2 hours while FT_4 reaches its highest
levels 24 hours after delivery. These increases in both T_4 and T_3
persist for 2-3 weeks while TSH levels return to normal within 2
days. It is, therefore, possible to evaluate the newborn for
hypothyroidism within 5-10 days of birth by measuring TSH.

SUGGESTED READING

Brennan MD: Thyroid hormones. Mayo Clin Proc 55:33, 1980

Burrow GN: The management of thyrotoxicosis in pregnancy. N Engl J
Med 313:562, 1985

Cooper DS: Antithyroid drugs. N Engl J Med 311:1353, 1984

Hamburger JI: The clinical spectrum of thyroiditis. Thyroid Today
3:1, 1980

Klein I, Levey GS: Thyroid storm. Hospital Medicine p34a, 1982

Vagenakis AG, Braverman LE, Azizi E, Portnay GI, Ingbar SH: Recovery of pituitary thyrotropic function after withdrawal of prolonged thyroid-suppression therapy. N Engl J Med 293:681, 1975

Van Herle AJ, Rich P, Ljung BE, Ashcraft MW, Solomon DH, Keeler EB: The thyroid nodule. Annals Int Med 96:221, 1982

Chapter 8

The Adrenal and Its Disorders

George A. Hill, M.D.

ADRENAL FUNCTION

Anatomy

The adrenal glands are paired pyramidal structures adhering to the upper poles of the kidneys. The adrenal cortex is divided into three zones.

Location	Name	Secretory Product
Outer	Zona Glomerulosa	Aldosterone
Mid	Zona Fasciculata	Corticosteroids
Inner	Zona Reticularis	Corticosteroids

Physiology

The adrenal cortex secretes mainly aldosterone, cortisol, and corticosterone, and small quantities of androgens. Aldosterone synthesis takes place in the zona glomerulosa and is dependent on changes in blood volume and in sodium-potassium balance. The renin angiotensin mechanism is most important in the control of aldosterone secretion. The adrenals of a normal, healthy, adult secrete approximately 25 mg of cortisol per day and the concentration of the steroid in the blood varies in a circadian pattern, associated with light-dark and sleep-wake cycles. The corticosteroids are synthesized from adrenal cholesterol (see Chapter 1) and are released into the circulation as soon as they are synthesized. Cortisol synthesis takes place in the zona fasciculata and zona reticularis and is dependent on pituitary adenocorticotrophin hormone (ACTH).

ACTH is a polypeptide composed of 39 amino acid residues. The N-terminal 1-24 amino acid sequence is essential for physiological activity, but the C-terminal 25-39 sequence is not. ACTH has a short half-life in blood. It is released rapidly in increased amounts in conditions of stress. The secretion of ACTH is controlled by corticotropin releasing factor (CRF, CRH) secreted in the hypothalamus and conveyed to the adenohypophysis by the hypothalamo-hypophyseal portal blood vessels. Vasopressin acts synergistically with CRF and is essential for the full expression of hypothalamo-pituitary-adenocorticotrophic activity. The activity of the CRF-producing neurons is under the control of afferent impulses from higher centers in the brain. The circadian rhythm in ACTH secretion is under the influence of afferent pathways different from those controlling the release of the hormone in response to stress. It appears that central cholinergic nervous pathways stimulate and that GABA-ergic and adrenergic pathways inhibit the secretion of CRF. The blood corticosteroid concentration is the major factor involved in the negative feedback effects on the secretion of corticotropin.

Effects of Corticosteroids

Because of the known effects of the corticosteroids, the result of either hypo- or hypersecretion can be predicted:

Decreased Cortisol

1. Increased sodium excretion and a decrease in plasma sodium
2. Plasma potassium increases
3. Blood volume decreases, peripheral vascular resistance decreases, and cardiac output and myometrial contractility decrease, leading to a decrease in the blood pressure
4. The urine cannot be concentrated or diluted
5. Liver and muscle glycogen are depleted
6. Fasting plasma glucose declines
7. Quantity of nonprotein nitrogen in the urine decreases

Increased Cortisol

1. Blood volume expands, and the blood pressure may rise
2. Plasma potassium falls
3. The excretion of nitrogen rises, leading to a negative nitrogen balance
4. Glycogen in liver, myocardium, and striated muscle is increased
5. Blood glucose may rise
6. Connective tissue is reduced in quantity and strength, and cell mediated immunity is impaired, leading to impaired inflammation and wound healing

Measurement of Adrenal Output and Function

1. ACTH: When adrenal hyperfunction has been established, plasma ACTH measurements will help to differentiate adrenal tumors from pituitary and ectopic sources of ACTH.

2. Glucocorticoids: The synthesis and secretion of cortisol is regulated by ACTH. Cortisol concentration is highest around 8:00 AM and lowest between 11:00 PM and 4:00 AM. Cortisol circulates bound to plasma proteins, the major one being cortisol binding globulin (CBG). Cortisol is 90% bound to CBG up to concentrations of 25 µg/dl, but as cortisol concentrations rise above this level, the binding capacity of CBG is exceeded and the proportion of free cortisol rises greatly. The synthesis of CBG is increased by estrogens, oral contraceptives, pregnancy and hyperthyroidism resulting in elevated serum cortisol concentrations. Circadian patterns must be kept in mind when interpreting the results of cortisol measurements.

3. Urinary Free Cortisol: Approximately 75-100 µg of free cortisol is secreted in the urine each day. This is a reliable means of assessing the adrenal glucocorticoid status especially when there is a question of cortisol excess. This test is preferable to the 17-OHCS because it correlates well with cortisol production rates and is not subject to color interference.

4. Urinary 17-Hydroxycorticosteroids (17-OHCS): The measurement of 17-OHCS represents a measure of predominantly cortisol metabolites secreted in the urine over 24 hours. However, the 24-hour 17-OHCS also includes other minor steroid subfractions, and therefore, is not a good index of steroid secretion or a reliable indicator of the biological activity of specific steroids. In fact, 24% of patients with Cushing's syndrome may not have increased excretion of 17-OHCS.

5. Dehydroepriandrosterone Sulfate (DHEA-S): This androgen is produced almost entirely by the adrenal gland. It can be measured by sensitive radioimmunoassay and is a good index of adrenal androgen function because of its stability and lack of fluctuation.

6. Urinary 17-Ketosteroids (17-KS): The 24-hour urinary 17-KS measure metabolites of steroids derived from both the adrenal cortex and the gonads. These are mainly a

measurement of androgens and their metabolites. Like the
17-OHCS, this is not a good index of steroid secretion
nor reliable indicator of the biological activity of
specific steroids secreted by the endocrine glands.
One-half of patients with polycystic ovarian syndrome who
have increased concentration of androstenedione and
testosterone have normal urinary excretion of 17-KS.

ADRENAL STIMULATION TESTS

   Stimulatory tests are needed to diagnosis adrenal problems
when static tests of adrenal function are nondiagnostic. These
tests are especially useful in a patient suspected of having adrenal
insufficiency.

   1. ACTH Stimulation: This test may be performed as a rapid
test (generally used as a screening test) or as a continuous ACTH
infusion test (which may be used as a diagnostic test). If the peak
cortisol is greater than or equal to 20 µg/dl then this suggests
normal adrenal function as assessed by the rapid ACTH test. The
increased rise in plasma cortisol in the normal patient will
generally be greater than 7 µg/dl. The time of day is not important
in the rapid ACTH test. It is performed as follows:

CORTROSYN STIMULATION

   a. Blood for plasma cortisol is drawn at time 0.
   b. Synthetic 1-24 ACTH (Cortrosyn) 0.25 mg is given IV.
   c. Blood for plasma cortisol is drawn at 30 and 60 minutes
      (the maximal rise in plasma cortisol occurs between
      30 and 60 minutes).

   If the rapid ACTH test is abnormal or borderline, then a 48-
hour continuous ACTH infusion test should be performed. This test
is performed as follows:

   a. A 24-hour urine is collected as baseline for urinary
      cortisol.
   b. Cortrosyn, 0.25 mg in 500 ml of saline, is infused over
      8 hours on 3 consecutive days.
   c. Concomitant 24-hour urine collections for urinary
      cortisol are performed.

   The demonstration of a normal response to ACTH shows the
presence of a responsive adrenal cortex, but it does not give

information about the ability of the pituitary to respond normally to physiological demands.

2. <u>CRF Stimulation Test</u>: The CRF stimulation test is used to test pituitary responsiveness directly. Ovine-CRF is given as a bolus intravenous injection (1 µg/kg). If the pituitary is responsive, a rise of ACTH will be noted within 2 minutes, and peak levels will be noted at 10-15 minutes. Plasma cortisol begins to rise at about 10 minutes and reaches its peak of at least 13 µg/dl at 30-60 minutes.

3. <u>Insulin-Induced Hypoglycemia</u>: This test measures the capacity of insulin-induced hypoglycemia to increase the concentration of cortisol and/or ACTH in plasma. The response to hypoglycemia is the most reliable of the various tests for the integrity of the hypothalamic-pituitary-adrenal system. The test is performed by injecting 0.15 units of regular insulin per kg of body weight. The maximal fall in blood glucose is achieved 30 minutes after insulin injection and should be 40 mg/dl or less. The normal plasma cortisol response at 45 minutes is a rise to 1.5 times the pretreatment level, a rise of at least 7 µg/dl, and a maximal level greater than 18 µg/dl. The maximal rise of ACTH is an increment of 3.5 times the preinjection level. This test should not be used in patients with known pituitary or adrenal insufficiency and a reduced dosage (0.1 unit/kg body weight) may be advisable in patients in whom the diagnosis seems highly likely. An ampule of 50% dextrose should be available for immediate use if necessary.

4. <u>Metyrapone Test</u>: Metyrapone inhibits 11β hydroxylase and, therefore, prevents cortisol and corticosterone synthesis, lowering their plasma levels. In normal individuals, this diminishes feedback inhibition and causes release of ACTH, which in turn stimulates the adrenal to activate steroid synthesis. Since cortisol cannot be produced because of the action of the drug, 11-deoxycortisol (Compound S) is the major product, and in normal individuals will increase 100 times the control level.

ADRENAL SUPPRESSION TESTS

1. <u>Overnight Dexamethasone Suppression Test</u>: This test is carried out by giving a single oral dose of 1 mg of dexamethasone at 11:00 PM, and measuring a plasma cortisol at 8:00 AM the following morning. In normal patients, the plasma cortisol level will be less than 5 µg/dl. This rapid test is useful for screening purposes, however, false positive tests do occur. Anyone with an abnormal result should have a low dose and/or high dose dexamethasone suppression test to arrive at a final diagnosis. However, there are factors which can alter the test results:

1. Phenytoin
2. Sympathomimetics and nasal decongestants
3. Oral contraceptive pills
4. Depression
5. Substantial weight loss
6. Chronic alcoholism
7. Hospitalized patients

2. Low and High Dose Dexamethasone Suppression: This test is carried out by measuring plasma levels of cortisol on the evening before and each morning of the test. A 0.5 mg dose of dexamethasone is then given orally every 6 hours for at least 2 days. After the initial suppression period, the dose is raised to 2.0 mg every 6 hours and the collections continued for 2 more days. In normal persons, the plasma cortisol should be below 5 μg/dl at 4:00 PM on the second day of the low-dose schedule. Patients who do not suppress on the low-dose schedule should have a value of less than 10 μg/dl at 4:00 PM on the second day of the high dose test if bilateral adrenal hyperplasia is present. Failure to suppress on high-dose dexamethasone suggests adrenal tumor (adenoma or carcinoma) or ectopic ACTH syndrome.

ADRENAL INSUFFICIENCY (ADDISON'S DISEASE)

Inadequate secretion of corticosteroid may occur as a result of insufficient secretion of ACTH or because of complete or partial destruction of the adrenal glands. Autoimmune destruction of the adrenal glands is found in 80% of patients presenting with Addison's disease.

Manifestations of Addison's disease may appear acutely with life-threatening collapse, or may develop so gradually and insidiously that the date of onset of the disease cannot be recognized. Etiological causes include:

Adrenal disease (primary)
    Autoimmune (idiopathic)
    Tuberculosis
    Metastatic cancer
    Hemorrhagic destruction

Pituitary or hypothalamic (secondary or tertiary)
    Tumor
    Infiltrative diseases (sarcoidosis)
    Postpartum hemorrhage (Sheehan's syndrome)

Acute Adrenal Insufficiency: Most cases of acute adrenal
insufficiency arise in patients with undiagnosed chronic adrenal
disease. Many patients will have an antecedent history suggestive
of prolonged adrenal insufficiency including weight loss, anorexia,
fatigue, dizziness, and possible darkening skin. Acute adrenal
insufficiency may also occur in patients with known adrenal
insufficiency who do not realize their need for additional steroids
during times of stress.

Symptoms include:
> Fever or hypothermia
> Anorexia, nausea, vomiting, abdominal pain
> Hypotension, shock
> Symptoms of precipitating illness

Laboratory findings include:
> Electrolytes
>> Hyponatremia
>> Hyperkalemia, though normo- or hypokalemia
>> frequent
>> Low plasma bicarbonate
>> High urinary sodium concentration
> Others
>> High blood urea nitrogen (BUN)
>> Low to normal plasma glucose
>> Low to "inappropriately normal" plasma cortisol

Diagnosis: The diagnosis of acute adrenal insufficiency is
clinical. Empiric corticosteroid therapy should be initiated
without waiting for the results of steroid studies. The diagnosis
is made by demonstrating a low baseline plasma cortisol with failure
of the plasma cortisol level to respond to exogenous administration
of ACTH. This can be performed as follows:

a. Obtain a 10-ml blood sample for baseline cortisol level.
b. Administer 0.25 mg of Cortrosyn (ACTH I-24) intravenously
   in 1 ml of normal saline.
c. Draw a blood sample for cortisol 60 minutes after
   injection of Cortrosyn.
d. Before the test, administer 8 mg of dexamethasone
   intravenously to cover the acute adrenal insufficiency.

The normal response would be an increase in the cortisol level
of at least 10 µg/dl or a 3-fold rise. Dexamethasone minimally
interferes with the cortisol assay. If the rapid ACTH stimulation
test is positive, then a prolonged ACTH stimulation test should be
performed at a later time. A patient should not be committed to

lifelong steroid replacement on the basis of a rapid ACTH
stimulation test.

Treatment:

1. Identify and treat the precipitating event
   a. Infection (viral or bacterial)
   b. Psychological stress
   c. Other stresses
2. Fluid and electrolyte therapy
   a. Fluid: Intravenous infusion of normal saline and
      dextrose until signs and symptoms of intravascular
      volume depletion are stabilized. Frequently, 5 liters
      or more are needed in the first 24 hours. Intravenous
      fluids are required until oral intake is stabilized.
   b. Potassium: Hyperkalemia frequently responds to volume
      expansion and hormonal replacement. Expect the
      potassium to drop with therapy; therefore plasma
      potassium must be monitored carefully and potassium
      given if hypokalemia occurs.
3. Hormonal replacement
   a. Give 200-300 mg intravenous injection of hydrocortisone
      (Solu-Cortef) immediately.
   b. Follow with 100 mg hydrocortisone intravenously every 8
      hours until stable.
   c. Give 50 mg cortisone acetate intramuscularly every 12
      hours until stable.
   d. After stabilization, decrease the dose of
      hydrocortisone 20-40% daily until maintenance therapy
      achieved.
   e. When the hydrocortisone dosage is reduced below 100-150
      mg daily fludrocortisone acetate may be needed.
4. Education of patient
   a. Increase (double) daily steroid dosage with minor
      stress until stress is alleviated.
   b. Wear Medic-Alert bracelet.
   c. Educate family members about adrenal insufficiency.

Chronic Adrenal Insufficiency: The clinical picture of full blown
chronic adrenocorticol insufficiency is easy to recognize, however,
the syndrome may develop so gradually that it is difficult to
recognize.

Symptoms	Signs
Weakness and easy fatigue	Loss of weight
Anorexia	Hyperpigmentation
Vomiting	Electrolyte disturbance
Constipation	Hypotension
Abdominal pain	Abnormal electroencephalogram
Diarrhea	Spontaneous hypoglycemia
Salt craving	Adrenal calcification
Muscle and joint pains	Vitiligo
Postural giddiness	

Diagnosis: Subtle laboratory abnormalities such as hypoglycemia, decreased sodium, or increased potassium levels may suggest the diagnosis of chronic adrenal insufficiency, however, the only way to diagnose this syndrome is to test the adrenal response to ACTH as previously described. It is unsafe to depend on a single determination of urinary or plasma steroids, however, a definite diagnosis of primary adrenal insufficiency can be made if the plasma cortisol is low at the same time that the plasma ACTH concentration is higher than normal.

Patients with primary adrenal insufficiency have no rise in the urinary cortisol during the long ACTH stimulation test whereas patients with secondary adrenal insufficiency will have a subnormal rise on the first day and will increase to three times the baseline by the third day. A shorter method using a 48-hour continuous infusion of Cortrosyn, 0.25 mg in 500 ml normal saline, every 12 hours is equally valid.

Treatment: Hydrocortisone, 20 mg each morning and 10 mg each evening, is usually effective. The dosage may be adjusted up or down based on the patients response. With this regimen, most patients will also require fludrocortisone, 0.05-0.1 mg, each day. This can be adjusted according to the blood pressure response as well as the serum potassium level. Patients with chronic adrenal insufficiency should be educated about their disease and should wear "Medic-Alert" bracelets. They must inform other health care professionals that they see of their disease, and should know to increase their dose of steroid in times of stress.

Patients with known adrenal insufficiency must be covered adequately for surgical procedures. This may be accomplished by administering cortisone acetate, 50-75 mg intramuscularly, the night before surgery and 100 mg of hydrocortisone intravenously on call to the operating room. During surgery, 100 mg of hydrocortisone should be infused continuously as needed. Postoperatively 100 mg of

hydrocortisone with dextrose and/or normal saline should be infused
continuously every 8 hours until the patient is stable. The steroid
dosage can then be decreased to maintenance levels.

During the last half of pregnancy, steroid requirements double,
therefore, pregnant patients with adrenal insufficiency must have
their dose of steroids increased appropriately. Mineralocorticoid
requirements may decrease secondary to the salt-retaining effects of
gestational steroids. At the time of delivery, the pregnant patient
should be managed similar to the surgical patient with adrenal
insufficiency. Steroid requirements drop rapidly after delivery.

GLUCOCORTICOID PREPARATIONS

USP Name	Trade Name	Relative anti-inflammatory Potency	Relative Mineralocorticoid Potency	Approximate Equivalent Dosage
Short acting				
Hydrocortisone (Cortisol)	Cortef Solu-Cortef	1.0	1.0	20.0
Cortisone		0.8	0.8	25.0
Prednisone	Deltasone Meticorten	4.0	0.8	5.0
Prednisolone	Delta-Cortef Meticortelone	4.0	0.8	5.0
Melthylprednisolone	Medrol Solu-medrol	5.0	0.5	4.0
Intermediate acting				
Triamcinolone	Aristocort Kenacort	5.0	0	4.0
Paramethasone	Haldrone	10.0	0	2.0
Long acting				
Dexamethasone	Decadron Hexcadrol	25.0	0	0.75
Betamethasone	Celestone	25.0	0	0.6

GLUCOCORTICOID EXCESS (CUSHING'S SYNDROME)

Cushing's syndrome results from the sum of the various
metabolic abnormalities induced by excessive amounts of
glucocorticoids, principally cortisol. The most common cause of
Cushing's syndrome is the use of pharmacological doses of potent
glucocorticoids for nonendocrine disorders.

The term Cushing's disease refers to adrenal hyperplasia
resulting from excessive secretion of pituitary ACTH. This
represents 70-80% of all cases of Cushing's syndrome. Cushing's
syndrome can also result from increased secretion of ACTH from
sources other than the pituitary (ectopic ACTH secretion) or from
increased secretion of glucocorticoids by adrenal adenomas or
carcinomas. Cushing's syndrome is nine times more common in females
than males.

CLINICAL MANIFESTATIONS OF CUSHING'S SYNDROME

Obesity (face, chin, supraclavicular fat pads, trunk, abdomen)	Easy bruising
	Hypertension
Wasting of the extremities	Hirsutism
Thin skin	Menstrual disorders
Facial plethora	Acne
Violaceous striae	Psychological disturbances
Muscle weakness	Hypokalemia
Back pain (2^0 to osteoporosis)	Metabolic alkalosis

Diagnosis: The diagnosis of hypercortisolism can be suspected based on the clinical history and findings from the physical examination. However, the diagnosis must be confirmed by specific tests of adrenal function.

1. Overnight dexamethasone test: This test as described previously is the easiest screening test to perform. A normal result excludes the diagnosis of Cushing's syndrome. Positive results must be followed by the low-dose or high-dose dexamethasone suppression test.

2. Urinary free cortisol: Typically, patients with hypercortisolism will secrete at least 125 µg of free cortisol in the urine per 24 hours. Serum cortisol determinations are not helpful.

3. CRF test: Patients with Cushing's disease (pituitary ACTH secretion) have increased blood levels of ACTH after injections of CRF. Patients with various forms of ectopic ACTH production do not have an elevation of ACTH after intravenous injection of CRF.

4. CT scan: A CT scan of the pituitary may be useful in identifying pituitary adenomas. CT scan of the adrenals may also be useful in identifying adrenal adenomas or carcinomas. CT scan of the chest looking for small tumors may be useful in patients who are suspected of having ectopic ACTH secretion (although chest x-ray should be performed first and may identify larger masses).

5. Catheterizaton of the inferior petrosal sinus to measure ACTH gradient if one needs to identify the pituitary as the source of ACTH.

6. **Serum ACTH:** This test may be helpful in differentiating syndromes of pituitary and ectopic secretion of ACTH from adrenal masses.

DIFFERENTIATION OF HYPERCORTISOLISM

	Urinary free Cortisol	Serum ACTH	Overnight Dexamethasone Suppression	High dose Dexamethasone Suppression	CRF Test
Pituitary ACTH secretion	↑	↑	No suppression	Suppression	↑ACTH
Ectopic ACTH secretion	↑	↑	No suppression	No suppression	No ↑ ACTH
Adrenal Adenoma	↑	↓	No suppression	No suppression	Blunted ACTH response

TREATMENT

The ideal therapy for any form of Cushing's syndrome should lower the daily cortisol secretion to normal, extirpate any tumor that might threaten the health of the patient, avoid lifelong endocrine deficiency, and avoid permanent dependence on medication. Several therapies are available, each decision made on the basis of the etiology of the hypercortisolism.

1. **Transsphenoidal Pituitary Surgery (TPS):** TPS can cure 85-90% of patients with pituitary adenomas while preserving pituitary function. Transient diabetes insipidus is the most common complication of TPS, other rare complications include meningitis, optic nerve damage, cerebrospinal fluid leak, and sinusitis. If hypocortisolism is not demonstrable immediately after TPS, then it is unlikely that the patient is cured even when the urinary cortisol level is normal and dexamethasone suppressibility can be demonstrated. Patients who are not cured by TPS fall into four groups:

a. Those with invasive pituitary tumor
b. Those with unidentified microadenomas
c. Those with corticotrope hyperplasia in the absence of a discrete adenoma
d. Those with ectopic production of corticotropin

2. <u>Adrenalectomy</u>: Bilateral adrenalectomy may be used in patients with hypercortisolism who do not respond to TPS. This offers an immediate and permanent means of reversing hypercortisolism. The disadvantages of bilateral adrenalectomy include significant perioperative mortality and mordidity, persistant or recurrent hypercortisolism due to adrenal tissue not removed at surgery, and Nelson's syndrome. Bilateral adrenalectomy is less appealing because of these complications.

3. <u>Pituitary irradiation</u>: Heavy-particle irradiation (8000 rad) can be given as a single treatment with multiple ports and usually results in high cure rates. Complications include hypopituitarism and ocular nerve palsy. Conventional cobalt 60 irradiation (5000 rad) can be used and is useful in children with Cushing's disease. No complications have been reported from this form of therapy. Cure rates for adults are only 15-20%, therefore, it is not useful in adults.

4. <u>Neuropharmacotherapeutic drugs</u>: These agents are only partially successful in decreasing excessive corticotropin secretion and must be considered adjunctive therapy.
   a. Serotonin antagonist - cyproheptadine: After administration for several months, approximately 50% of patients with Cushing's disease are helped, serum cortisol and corticotropin levels normalize and there is a return of normal dexamethasone suppressibility in some patients. As soon as cyproheptadine is withdrawn, hypercortisolism generally returns. Side-effects include hyperphagia, weight gain, and sommolence.
   b. Dopamine agonist - bromocriptine: Approximately one-half of patients with Cushing's syndrome will suppress their secretion of corticotropin with bromocriptine administration. However, very few patients actually decrease their cortisol secretion to the normal range.
   c. Norepinephrine depletion - Reserpine: Preliminary studies using small doses of reserpine (0.25 mg every 8 hours) show that some patients have complete remission of Cushing's disease.
   d. Gamma-Aminobutyric Acid (GABA) Antagonist - Valproate Sodium: GABA is an inhibitory neurotransmitter which has been demonstrated to be involved in corticosteroid feedback and CRF release in the rat. Valproate sodium decreases corticotropin secretion. Corticotropin secretion generally returns to pretreatment levels once the drug is discontinued.

Cushing's Syndrome in Pregnancy

Maternal complications in patients with Cushing's syndrome are quite common. Almost one-half of patients with an adrenal adenoma will develop pulmonary edema, and almost all patients where pregnancy progresses to the first trimester experience hypertension. Maternal complications are much less common in patients with adrenal hyperplasia. There is a high incidence of prematurity. Early diagnosis and prompt treatment of patients with Cushing's syndrome is of vital importance.

INCIDENTAL ADRENAL MASS

Benign, clinically silent, adrenal adenomas have been found to be present in 1.4-8.7% of patients undergoing autopsy. Since only a very rare occult nonfunctioning adrenocortical carcinoma will be found, an approach to management of these lesions is needed. Furthermore, with the increasing frequency of CT scans of the abdomen being utilized, more and more of these masses will be discovered.

ADRENAL MASSES IN ADULTS

Cortical adenomas	Cysts
Cortical carcinomas	Myelolipomas
Pheochromocytomas	Adenolipomas
Ganglioneuromas	Mestastases from other tumors

Evaluation of the Adrenal Mass

Determination of the biochemical activity is a fundamental consideration in the assessment of adrenal masses. Other factors which need to be evaluated include the age and sex of the patient, the size of the mass, its imaging characteristics, and its cytological features. A thorough search should be made for evidence of Cushing's syndrome, virilization, feminization, mineralocorticoid excess, and catecholamine excess. A primary adrenal malignancy may show evidence of local extension or distant metastasis, most commonly to lung, liver, lymph nodes, peritoneum, bone, and pelvis. Metastases to the adrenal gland from nonadrenal tumors should also be considered.

Although women outnumber men 6:1 with Cushing's syndrome, men outnumber women 2:1 among patients with clinically nonfunctional carcinomas. Older patients have a higher incidence of endocrinologically silent carcinomas.

LABORATORY ASSESSMENT

Urinary free cortisol
Urinary 17-ketosteroids
Low-dose dexamethasone suppression test
Plasma testosterone (if virilism or
  hirsutism present in a female or child)
Plasma estrogen (if feminization present in
  a male or child)
Serum potassium
Metanephrines, catecholamines, and/or
  vanillylmandelic acid

The CT scan offers the most promise in imaging adrenal masses. Plain film of the abdomen and arteriography are of no great benefit. Ultrasound may be useful in these patients, but generally is not helpful. Fine needle aspiration of an adrenal mass is most helpful in the differential diagnosis of a cystic mass. Clear fluid signals a benign cyst. Bloody fluid may be associated with a benign or malignant lesion. Cytological evaluation of fine needle aspirates holds little promise.

SUGGESTED READING

Carpenter PC: Cushing's syndrome: update of diagnosis and management. Mayo Clin Proc 61:49, 1986

Chamberlin P, Meyer WJ: Management of pituitary-adrenal suppression secondary to corticosteroid therapy. Pediatrics 67:245, 1981

Chrousos GP, Schuermeyer TH, Doppman J, Oldfield EH, Schulte HM, Gold PW, Loriaux DL: Clinical applications of corticotropin-releasing factor. Ann Intern Med 102:344, 1985

Copeland PM: The incidentally discovered adrenal mass. Ann Intern Med 98:940, 1983

Hamburger S, Rush D: Series on endocrine metabolic emergencies: II. acute adrenal insufficiency. JAMWA 36:199, 1981

Hodges JR: The hypothalamo-pituitary-adrenocortical system. Br J Anaesth 56:701, 1984

May ME, Carey RM: Rapid adrenocorticotropic hormone test in practice. Am J Med 79:679, 1985

Chapter 9

Dysmenorrhea and Premenstrual Syndrome

George A. Hill, M.D.

DYSMENORRHEA

DEFINITION

Dysmenorrhea commonly refers to painful menstruation. It may be primary dysmenorrhea or secondary dysmenorrhea depending on the presence or absence of pelvic pathology.

INCIDENCE

Over 50% of menstruating women are affected by dysmenorrhea, and about 10% of women with dysmenorrhea are severely affected or incapacited for 1-3 days each month.

ETIOLOGY

There is evidence that increased production and release of endometrial prostaglandins during menstruation may be responsible for the uterine cramps in many women with primary dysmenorrhea. The systemic symptoms listed are well known side-effects of the administration of PGE_2 or $PGF_2\alpha$, and therefore, may also be related to the endometrial release of prostaglandins during menstruation. It is also known that secretory endometrium contains higher concentrations of prostaglandins, consistent with the theory that primary dysmenorrhea occurs only in ovulatory cycles.

At the end of the luteal phase of the menstrual cycle, if the patient is not pregnant, progesterone declines as the corpus luteum regresses. This decrease in progesterone leads to lysosomal instability. Menstruation begins and phospholipase A_2 is released leading to hydrolysis of phospholipids from the cell membrane and generation of arachidonic acid, the precursor of the prostaglandins.

The availability of phospholipase A_2 is the rate limiting step in the synthesis of PGE_2 and $PGF_{2\alpha}$, therefore, once arachidonic acid is available, synthesis of PGE_2 and $PGF_{2\alpha}$ proceeds rapidly. These prostaglandins then produce local symptoms such as uterine cramping as well as the systemic symptoms listed.

Menstrual fluid prostaglandins have been measured and are significantly higher in women with dysmenorrhea compared to normal women. Other factors such as behavioral and psychological factors, or increased vasopressin release may also be related to dysmenorrhea.

CLINICAL FEATURES

Primary Dysmenorrhea:

1. The pain occurs almost invariably in ovulatory cycles.
2. It usually appears 6-12 months after menarche when ovulatory cycles are established.
3. It usually begins several hours before or just after the onset of menstruation and lasts for 48-72 hours.
4. The pain is most severe on the first day. It is spasmodic in nature, stronger over the lower abdomen, and described as crampy or labor-like.
5. In over 50% of patients with dysmenorrhea, the pelvic pain is accompanied by one or more systemic symptoms. These include:

Nausea and vomiting	89%
Fatigue	85%
Diarrhea	60%
Lower backache	60%
Headaches	45%

6. The pelvic examination is normal.

Secondary Dysmenorrhea:

1. Symptoms begin to occur remote from menarche, and are similar to those noted in primary dysmenorrhea.
2. The most frequent cause is pelvic endometriosis.
3. In patients with anovulatory cycles the dysmenorrhea is usually secondary.

Likely causes include:
  Endometriosis
  Intrauterine device
  Acute or chronic salpingitis
  Other pelvic infections

Less common causes include:
  Uterine myomas
  Polyps
  Adhesions
  Congenital malformations of the mullerian system
  Cervical stricture or stenosis
  Ovarian cysts
Rare causes include:
  Pelvic congestion syndrome
  Allen-Master's syndrome

INVESTIGATION

The initial investigation for primary or secondary dysmenorrhea should include:

1. A complete history, general physical examination, and pelvic examination.
2. Complete blood count and erythrocyte sedimentation rate should be obtained to establish a diagnosis of acute or chronic pelvic infection or inflammation.
3. Cervical culture for gonorrhea, chlamydia, and/or ureaplasma may be helpful to establish the diagnosis of a pelvic infection.
4. If urinary symptoms are present, urine analysis and/or urine culture may be needed.
5. A hysterosalpingogram (HSG) will help establish the diagnosis of mullerian abnormalities. An ultrasonogram may be needed to delineate further abnormalities found during the pelvic examination or laboratory evaluation.

Further Work Up:

1. A laparoscopy may be helpful in the definitive diagnosis of mullerian abnormalities or to establish the diagnosis of pelvic pathology such as endometriosis, pelvic adhesions, ovarian cysts, etc.
2. Hysteroscopy may be helpful in diagnosing or treating mullerian abnormalities.
3. D & C may be helpful in relieving the symptoms of dysmenorrhea in a small percentage of patients.

THERAPY

Primary Dysmenorrhea:

Prostaglandin synthetase inhibitors (PGSI) are the first choice in the therapy of dysmenorrhea, especially if the patient does not need contraception. These drugs relieve dysmenorrhea by:
Inhibition of cyclic endoperoxide synthesis
Blockage of cyclic endoperoxide cleavage enzyme

If the PGSI does not relieve the dysmenorrhea, or in the patient desiring contraception, oral contraceptive pills (OCP) should be added to the regimen. OCPs relieve dysmenorrhea by:
Decreasing menstrual fluid prostaglandin concentrations
Decreasing menstrual fluid volume
Suppression of ovulation

Clinical Group	Derivative	Brand Name	Dosage
Arylpropionic acid	Ibuprofen	Motrin	400 mg QID
	Naproxen sodium	Anaprox	275 mg QID
		Naprosyn	275 mg QID
Fenamates	Mefenamic acid	Ponstel	250-500 mg QID
		Meclomen	50-100 mg QID
Indol-acetic acid	Indomethacin	Indocin	25-50 mg TID
Buterophenone	Phenylbutazone	Butazolidin	100 mg QID
Benzoic acid	Acetylsalicylic acid	Aspirin	625 mg QID

Therapeutic Agents Useful in the Treatment of Dysmenorrhea

If the response to PGSIs or OCPs is unsatisfactory, laparoscopy is indicated to evaluate the pelvis for other pathology which might be etiological in the symptomatology.

Secondary Dysmenorrhea:

After treating the underlying cause, other methods of treatment should also include the use of PSGIs and OCPs if no other contraindication exists for their use. Conservative medical therapy should always be attempted first, since surgical therapy may not improve the pain, and may make the pain worse. However, surgery should not be postponed indefinitely. Patients who do not respond to medical therapy need surgical therapy for both diagnosis and treatment.

Presacral neurectomy is indicated if there is:

1. Chronic pelvic pain with failure of other medical and surgical therapies.
2. Other pelvic pathology present with pain mediated by the presacral plexis.

Psychiatric consultation should be considered if:

1. The patient continues to complain of disabling pain or demands narcotics despite inhibition of ovulation and lack of evidence of endometriosis or another cause of secondary dysmenorrhea.
2. The patient refuses to permit a minimal examination or is unable to give a coherent history.
3. There are obvious emotional problems such as family disturbances, depression, gross social maladjustment, history of running away, alcohol abuse, drug abuse, or criminal behavior.
4. There is a suspicion of forced incest or sexual abuse.

CONCLUSION

Dysmenorrhea can be a complex problem for the practicing gynecologist. While the majority of patients will respond to conservative treatment and support, those who do not may require laparoscopy to determine if other pelvic factors are responsible for the dysmenorrhea. In certain situations psychiatric consultation may be a useful adjunct to therapy.

PREMENSTRUAL SYNDROME

INTRODUCTION

Frank published the first description of "premenstrual tension" in 1931. Over the next 20 years, very little was added since most clinicians believed this to be a psychosomatic disorder. In 1953, Green and Dalton changed the terminology to "premenstrual syndrome" (PMS) to allow the inclusion of additional somatic and psychological complaints. Since the late 1970s increased public and scientific scrutiny of PMS has prompted a re-evaluation of this syndrome. Over 150 symptoms have been listed as possible premenstrual complaints.

DEFINITION

Sutherland and Stewart defined PMS as any combination of emotional or physical signs or symptoms which occur cyclically prior to menstruation and regress or disappear after menstruation. When symptoms occur and interfere with normal daily function in a cyclical pattern conforming to the above definitions, most investigators agree with the label PMS.

INCIDENCE

Any woman with cyclic ovarian function can have PMS. The presence of a uterus is not required. Premenstrual symptoms have been described in 15-100% of women of reproductive age, depending on the severity and type of symptoms examined, with the peak occurrence in the third and fourth decades of life.

Retrospective analyses indicate that 20-40% of American women complain of premenstrual symptoms at least moderate in severity, associated with some or all of their menstrual periods. Five to ten percent of women become severely affected at some point in their lives. This represents a significant segment of the population.

ETIOLOGY

Numerous etiologies have been proposed for the symptom complex of PMS. Behavioral phenomena as well as sensory or cognitive parameters have been found to vary with the phase of the menstrual cycle making it difficult to decide what might be etiological in PMS and what might be a normal part of the menstrual cycle.

Hypotheses Proposed for PMS

Ovarian Hormones: Several reports have linked PMS with inadequate corpus luteum function. A correlation of progesterone levels with PMS symptoms has been attempted. Progesterone is released in a pulsatile manner so that single or even multiple progesterone samples may not be reliable indicators of overall corpus luteum function. Various authors have reported both a decrease or an increase in progesterone levels in women with PMS. Other authors have demonstrated a correlation of estrogen levels with irritability and anxiety. Animal research has demonstrated behavioral effects mediated by estrogen which may be counteracted by progesterone. In addition, progesterone appears to have sedating properties. Other studies have shown that the progestins may be responsible for the provocation of the cyclical symptoms of PMS. Suppression of ovulation remains one of the effective modalities for treatment of PMS in some patients.

Endogenous Opiates: Decreases in peripheral levels of endogenous opiates have been identified in a subgroup of PMS patients. Endorphins can inhibit production of biogenic amines which may, in turn, produce changes in mood, increased appetite, and thirst. In the follicular phase of the cycle, levels of β endorphines are similar in patients with PMS and control patients. While β endorphines increase in the late luteal phase of control patients, the levels in PMS patients decrease and are significantly less than those seen in control patients.

Vitamin and Mineral Deficiencies: Estrogen may induce a relative deficiency of pyridoxine (vitamin B_6) which is important in the biosynthesis of dopamine and serotonin. Therefore, a decline in vitamin B_6 in the brain could produce symptoms of PMS. Studies have shown an improvement in PMS when treated with vitamin B_6 during the luteal phase. However, other studies have not found vitamin B_6 to be superior to placebo. Deficiencies in minerals such as magnesium have also been suggested as a potential cause of PMS.

Mineralocorticoid Hypothesis: PMS is often associated with bloating and fluid retention. Many authors think that corticoids may be etiological in PMS. Clinical studies have been unable to demonstrate any significant difference in aldosterone levels in women with PMS compared to normal controls. Metabolites of progesterone may be important in the etiology of fluid retention in patients with PMS.

Psychological: PMS symptoms appear to be exacerbated by stress, however, somatic factors may be secondary to hormonal alterations. The psychic factors may follow these biochemical and physical changes.

Androgen Hypothesis: Androgens may be associated with aggression. However, no good data demonstrate an association of increased androgens with PMS.

Hypoglycemia: No significant difference in glucose, insulin, or glucagon levels has been demonstrated in either the follicular or luteal phase in normal women or women with PMS.

Monoamine Neurotransmitters: Decreased neurotransmission of biogenic amines (norepinephrine and dopamine) has been implicated in the pathogenesis of depression. Increase in these amines has also been linked to psychosis, aggression, and irritability. In spite of this, no difference has been noted in peripheral venous concentrations of these neurotransmitters or their metabolites in women with PMS.

Prolactin: Conflicting studies demonstrate both normal and increased prolactin levels in PMS sufferers.

Prostaglandins: $PGF_{2\alpha}$ and PGE_2 are increased during the luteal phase. No clear link between the prostaglandins and PMS has been reported.

Allergies: Hypersensitivity to various substances is reportedly increased in some women prior to menses. An autoimmune allergic reaction to progesterone has been suggested as one possible etiology for PMS.

DIAGNOSIS

The diagnosis of PMS relies on the patient's subjective reporting of symptoms. Retrospective measures currently in use include the Moos Menstrual Distress Questionnaire, the 19 Symptom Questionnaire of Abraham, and the Premenstrual Assessment Form of Halbreich and Endicott. Since retrospective questionnaires are poor, the best way to establish whether a patient's complaints are cyclic (and thus referable to PMS) is to utilize a prospective, daily self-assessment form with an estimation of relative symptom severity.

A pooled 3-day sample for measuring progesterone (P_4) and estradiol (E_2) may be helpful in guiding therapy in patients thought to have PMS. We currently measure E_2 and P_4 in a pooled sample taken on ideal cycle days 20, 21, and 22. The ratio of $P_4:E_2$ is probably more important than the absolute values.

Other hormonal parameters may be measured if indicated from the findings of the physical examination. For example, a prolactin is needed if galactorrhea is present, and DHEAS and testosterone are needed if there are signs of hyperandrogenism.

TREATMENT ALTERNATIVES

Nonpharmacologic

Exercise: Clinical studies have demonstrated a reduction in anger, depression, and tension in women who exercise. Exercise is beneficial to the general health of the patient as well as the PMS symptoms.

Nutrition: Commonly recommended alterations in diet include a reduction in caffeine and a reduction in refined sugars. Frequent

small meals have been suggested for women with symptoms consistent
with reactive hypoglycemia.

Pharmacologic

Placebo: Placebos improve symptoms in up to 60% of subjects,
which makes objective assessment of pharmacologic modalities
difficult.

Progesterone: Only one randomized, double-blind, cross-over
trial has demonstrated that progesterone may be more efficacious in
reducing symptoms of PMS than placebo. In this study, 300 mg/day
of micronized P_4 was used and compared to placebo. The results
indicated significant improvement of anxiety, depression, stress,
swelling, and hot flushes with treatment. Maximum improvement was
noted during the first month of P_4 therapy. Numerous other studies
have been unable to demonstrate an improvement with P_4 over that
seen with placebo. However, patients with a low midluteal serum
P_4 level (low $P_4:E_2$ ratio), or a normal midluteal serum P_4 and high
midluteal serum E_2 (low $P_4:E_2$ ratio), may benefit from P_4
supplementation. No serious side-effects of P_4 have been reported.
However, minor complaints such as moniliasis, infection, rash,
flatulence, and abdominal cramping may occur. In addition, oral
P_4 may cause dizziness or sleepiness.

Synthetic Progestins: Controlled studies have failed to show
superiority of synthetic progestins over placebo.

Ovulation Suppression: Ovulation suppression has been
attempted in order to inhibit the marked fluctuation in estrogen and
progesterone in a normal ovulatory cycle.

GnRH: Therapy with GnRH agonist has been shown to
effectively attenuate the cyclic symptoms of PMS in a
selected group of patients. However, longterm therapy with
GnRH is impractical due to the effects of vasomotor
instability (hot flashes) and hypoestrogenism (atrophic
vagina, osteroporosis).

Danocrine: Several studies have shown improvement in
breast complaints in women with PMS. However, there has been
no real improvement in other symptoms. Side-effects and
expense make this an impractical approach to the long-term
treatment of women with PMS.

Oral Contraceptives: OCPs may be useful if no side-effects
are produced and if this method of birth control is acceptable

to the patient. However, some women with PMS note an exacerbation of symptoms with combination OCPs. Medroxyprogesterone acetate, 10 mg, or Norethindrone acetate, 5 mg daily, can inhibit ovulation in many women, suppress menses, and eliminate marked cyclic ovarian hormone variation, however, their side-effects may be difficult to differentiate from symptoms of PMS.

Bromocriptine: Several studies report clinical improvement in both affective and physical symptoms in PMS patients treated with bromocriptine. However, other studies have been unable to demonstrate any efficacy. Bromocriptine appears to be most effective in relieving breast symptoms.

Lithium: Double-blind, placebo-controlled, cross-over studies have shown no significant difference between lithium and placebo in patients with PMS.

Diuretics:

Spironolactone: Because of its diuretic and antiandrogenic properties, this drug is theoretically applicable to women with fluid retention or symptoms of androgen excess during the premenstruum. One study has shown that spironolactone, 25 mg, administered four times daily on days 18-26 of the menstrual cycle resulted in a significant improvement in global mood assessment and reduction of weight. Lower doses have been ineffective.

Other Diuretics: In women who gain weight during the premenstrual period other diurectics may prove effective by decreasing edema, breast swelling, abdominal swelling, irritability, depression, tension, nervousness, and anxiety.

Pyridoxine: Uncontrolled studies have shown an improvement in physical and affective symptoms in women on pyridoxine, 500 mg daily. A controlled study, however, was unable to demonstrate any significant benefit of pyridoxine, 50 mg daily, in women with PMS and depression. Doses above 500 mg of pyridoxine daily may cause a peripheral neuropathy.

Prostaglandin Antagonist and Precursors: Variable results have been reported with prostaglandin synthetase inhibitors. One study reported a significant improvement in irritability, depression, tension, abdominal pain, and headache with prostaglandin inhibitors. Prostaglandin inhibitors may be useful for emotional and somatic symptoms, however they are of no benefit in treating breast symptoms. PGSI inhibit not only PGF but also PGE. PGE_1 is thought to be beneficial in relieving many of the symptoms associated with PMS, therefore inhibition of this prostaglandin would be detrimental to PMS sufferers. In fact, substances containing gamma-linolenic acid (a precursor of PGE) may be given in an attempt to increase concentrations of PGE. Efamol is marketed for this purpose.

CONCLUSION:

1. No single treatment has proven effective for the treatment of PMS.
2. Diet and exercise counseling may result in improvement for some women and is an easy therapeutic modality.
3. Frequent follow up is required to provide both emotional support and the opportunity to assess symptoms and response to therapy.
4. Daily symptom diaries are important in the prospective evaluation of patients with PMS.
5. Baseline psychological screening should be performed on all women being evaluated for PMS.
6. When a woman's symptoms are not cyclic in nature and span the entire month, further psychiatric evaluation may be needed to differentiate patients with depression from those with PMS.
7. Therapy directed at the major complaint may be all that is needed in some patients.

SUGGESTED READING

Abraham GE: Nutritional factors in the etiology of the premenstrual tension syndromes. J Reprod Med 28:446, 1983

Abraham GE: Premenstrual tension. Current Problems in Obstetrics and Gynecology 3-39, Year Book Medical Publisher, Inc., Chicago, 1981

Abraham GE, Hargrove JT: Effect of vitamin B_6 on premenstrual symptomology in women with premenstrual tension syndromes: a double-blind cross-over study. Infertility 3:155, 1986

Chan WY, Dawood MY, Fuchs F: Prostaglandins in primary dysmenorrhea. Am J Med 70:535, 1981

Chuong CJ, Coulam CB, Kao PC, Bergstralh EJ, Go VLW: Neuropeptide levels in premenstrual syndrome. Fertil Steril 44:760, 1985

124

Dalton K: Diagnosis and clinical features of premenstrual syndrome.
In: Premenstrual Syndrome and Dysmenorrhea, MY Dawood, GL McGuire,
and LM Demers (eds), Baltimore-Munich, Urban Schwarzenberg, 1985,
page 13

Dawood MY: Choosing the correct therapy for dysmenorrhea.
Contemp Ob/Gyn 19:235, 1982

Dawood MY: Dysmenorrhea. J Reproduc Med 30:154, 1985

Dawood MY: Etiology and treatment of dysmenorrhea. Sem Reproduc
Endocrinol 3:283, 1985

DeJong R, Rubinow DR, Roy-Byrne P, Hoban MC, Grover GN, Post RM:
Premenstrual mood disorder and psychiatric illness. Am J Psychiatry
142:1359, 1985

Frank HT: The hormonal causes of premenstrual tension. Arch Neurol
Psychiatry 26:2053, 1931

Goei GS, Abraham GE: Effect of a nutritional supplement, Optivite,
on symptoms of premenstrual tension. J Reproduc Med 28:527, 1983

Chapter 10

Management of the Menopause

Anne Colston Wentz, M.D.

INTRODUCTION

One-third of a woman's life is spent postmenopause. Problems during the climacteric and afterward are unique, and management should begin as much as 15 years before anticipated menopause. A number of somatic, physiologic and psychologic changes occur, some of which are due to estrogen deficiency and others which are caused by the estrogen-independent consequences of aging.

DEFINITION

The climacteric is defined as that phase in the aging process of women marking the transition from the reproductive to the nonreproductive stage of life. It encompasses that period of time during which ovarian function waxes and wanes. It may be a period of varied and diverse symptomatology for some but not all women.

The menopause is defined as the last menstrual period, and is diagnosed in retrospect when a year without menses has elapsed. The average age of menopause is approximately 51 years, although surgical castration or premature menopause may make this occur years earlier.

ENDOCRINE CHANGES IN THE MENOPAUSE

During the climacteric, there is progressive loss of ovarian follicles until functional oocytes and their surrounding steroid-producing cells are no longer present. The climacteric is therefore characterized by less frequent ovulatory cycles and less sex hormone secretion. Ovarian estradiol (E_2) output decreases, androgen secretion becomes predominant, and estrone becomes the main circulating estrogen, due to peripheral conversion. The ovary decreases in size and becomes fibrotic. Hyperplasia of the hilus cells occurs, and these cells may have some androgen-producing capacity.

Oophorectomy in the postmenopausal women results in a further decrease of plasma testosterone, androstenedione, E_2 and estrone in the peripheral circulation, indicating that the postmenopausal ovary is not entirely inactive. The postmenopause is clearly associated with estrogen deprivation, although the ovary makes a small contribution of E_2 to the circulation. The adrenal supplies most of the androgen precursors for aromatization following the menopause, so the peripheral conversion of androstenedione to estrone and testosterone to E_2 accounts for some circulating estrogen. Adipose tissue is quantitatively the most important body site in aromatizing androgen to estrogen in the postmenopausal woman. Androstenedione secreted principally from the adrenal cortex is the substrate for estrone production by adipose tissue. Increasing body weight and age are both associated with an increased conversion of androstenedione to estrone. Estrogen deficiency causes a number of problems for the post-menopausal woman, whereas other changes are related to aging and are not estrogen-dependent.

Postmenopausal Signs and Symptoms
Related to Estrogen Deficiency

Definitely Related	Probably Related	Possibly Related
Amenorrhea	Atherosclerotic cardiovascular disease	Psychosexual
Vasomotor instability	Blood lipid changes	
Osteoporosis, Type I		
Genito-urinary atrophy		

Menopause symptoms can be related to (1) estrogen deprivation, or (2) senescence and aging. Symptoms definitely due to estrogen deficiency include the hot flash, and vaginal atrophy with dryness; osteoporosis is a disease of estrogen deprivation which develops later in life. Amenorrhea, atrophy of the skin, and urethritis are also estrogen-dependent. Psychologic problems including depression are indirectly related to estrogen deficiency; atherosclerotic vascular disease is associated with the decreased high density lipoprotein (HDL), and increased cholesterol and triglycerides characteristic of the menopause. Menopause symptoms which are estrogen-independent include osteoarthritis, and some psychosexual changes.

DIAGNOSIS OF THE MENOPAUSE

The combination of amenorrhea or significant oligoamenorrhea
with hot flashes is indicative of the menopausal status. A serum
β-hCG should be drawn to rule out pregnancy. FSH levels greater
than 40 mIU/ml on at least 3 occasions 4 weeks apart will make the
diagnosis.

EVALUATION OF THE CLIMACTERIC, PERIMENOPAUSAL PATIENT

MANAGEMENT OF THE CLIMACTERIC WOMAN

History: Menstrual   Sexual/psychosexual
            Medical/surgical   Family
                                          Lifestyle

Physical: BP, weight and height
           Breasts
           Pelvic

Laboratory Screening: complete blood count (CBC)   chemistries
                       urinalysis   lipid panel

Specific testing:

breast   mammography and/or thermography: yearly

cervix   PAP: 1-3 years

uterus   endometrial biopsy or brush: before hormone
               replacement therapy
            aspiration cytology: ? yearly

ovary   bimanual; ultrasonography: yearly

bone   dual photon absorptiometry: before therapy
            serum calcium, phosphorus
            urine calcium: creatinine ratio

The History

The history of a climacteric woman should include attention to
preventive medicine plus questioning about risk factors, nutrition,
and general health. The patient should be allowed to tell her story
concerning symptoms. A menstrual history is important to evaluate
for signs and symptoms of endometrial hyperplasia, including
breakthrough bleeding or spotting or menorrhagia. The patient's
mental and emotional status, and her degree of depression, should be

ascertained. Ask about symptoms of liver or gall bladder disease, and obtain a complete health history of breast or gynecologic diseases.

A family history of osteoporosis, arteriosclerotic cardiovascular disease, gynecologic or breast carcinomas, diabetes, obesity, infertility, and/or endometriosis should be ascertained.

The patient's lifestyle should be investigated. What are her nutritional and exercise habits, does she indulge in hard physical activity, does she smoke or eat junk foods, what is her sexual activity, has her weight been stable, and what menopausal symptoms interfere with the lifestyle she has chosen?

Physical Examination

Blood pressure and pulse measurements are needed.

Nutritional status is ascertained and the ideal body weight is compared to actual. Note the patients' general appearance, does she look healthy and happy, or not? Skin color and texture may be revealing. Is there evidence of hirsutism or hair loss?

The height and weight, plus crown-to-pubis and pubis-to-heel measurements should be included. The crown-to-pubis measurement of the normal premenopausal woman should be within 1 inch of the pubis-to-heel measurement. If the crown-to-pubis figure is at least 1.5 inches below the pubis-to-heel figure, bone has been lost in the upper spinal column.

Evaluate for asymmetric thyroid growth, nodularity, and goiter.

Evaluate for breast abnormalities, heart murmurs or cardiac enlargement; examine the abdomen for masses, hepatomegaly, or tenderness.

Pelvic Examination

A complete and satisfactory pelvic examination delineates uterine size and shape, adnexal structures and the cul-de-sac. A PAP smear is done, and endometrial sampling is required before treatment is started. If the examination is unsatisfactory because of vaginal stenosis, mucosal dryness, or obesity, then an ultrasound may be indicated to detect uterine fibroids, adnexal masses, or other pathology particularly if the ovaries have been retained following hysterectomy.

Other Baseline Investigations

Further evaluation should include a screening blood chemistry,
lipid profile, calcium and phosphorus to rule out hyperparathy-
roidism, and liver function tests.

A chest film is not always a useful screening test. An EKG may
be indicated. A baseline mammogram is indicated between ages 35 and
40 and is suggested yearly in any woman past the age of 45; with
self-examination of the breasts, this provides early detection for
most breast pathology. Exceptions are those with a family history
of breast cancer or previous breast cancer in the patient; these
women should have more frequent mammography. Pelvic ultrasonography
may be indicated and helpful.

Several types of bone densitometry measurements are available,
and may be useful in some women. Mass screening of pre- and
perimenopausal women for detection of those likely to develop
osteoporosis is neither cost-effective nor prognostic. The use of
diagnostic bone densitometry or CT scanning should be reserved for
the woman in whom the diagnosis of osteoporosis is uncertain, or in
the woman under therapy in whom evaluation of therapy is important.

DEVELOPMENT OF A TREATMENT PLAN

The decision must be made whether it is necessary to treat
peri- and postmenopausal women with what and for how long. Risk
factors must therefore have been evaluated. Indications for, and
relative and absolute contraindications to, various forms of therapy
must be ascertained.

INDICATIONS FOR ESTROGEN REPLACEMENT THERAPY

1. Vasomotor symptoms
2. Genitourinary atrophy
3. Osteoporosis prophylaxis

BENEFITS OF ESTROGEN REPLACEMENT THERAPY

Vasomotor Symptoms: The characteristic hot flash is described
as a feeling of intense heat beginning in the core of the body,
rising to the chest and face and later extending to the extremities.
A generalized total body warmth or sweat may be indicative of
hyperthyroidism; facial flushing may indicate pheochromocytoma. The
hot flash is so typical that it is usually distinguishable from
other types of feelings of heat or sweating.

Uncomfortable and embarassing symptomatology characterized by the hot flash should be treated. The hot flash affects 75-85% of women, about 82% for more than 1 year and about 25% for more than 5 years. Estrogen replacement therapy (ERT) is effective in most women. The "rule of thumb" with estrogen replacement is to use the lowest dose which is effective. In general, a regimen of conjugated estrogen 1.25 mg, calendar days 1-25, and medroxyprogesterone acetate 10 mg, calendar days 16-25, is effective and well-tolerated; other ERT regimens are discussed later.

Progestins can be shown to alter hot flash frequency and are effective alone in many but not all women. Other agents which have had some effectiveness in some studies include: clonidine, placebo, tranquilizers, sedatives, and propranolol. Estrogen replacement will always cure the hot flash, although the dosage and route of administration may need to be varied.

Genitourinary dryness and atrophy: Dyspareunia, vaginal dryness, mucosal abrasion and secondary bleeding and stenosis are indications for treatment of vaginal atrophy; dysuria, urinary frequency and urgency, and urge incontinence may also be improved by ERT. Vaginal dryness may be effectively treated by local application of an estrogen vaginal cream, daily for a week, followed by use 2-3 times a week. Vaginal absorption of estrogen is rapid, and if there are contraindications to estrogen usage, these apply to the vaginal route as well.

Osteoporosis. Peak bone mass occurs at age 35 years. As women age, they lose 1-3% of bone mass per year after menopause. At age 80 years, 30-50% has been lost. Vertebral compression fractures occur in 25% of women over age 60 years and 50% of women over age 75 years. These cause chronic back pain, loss of height, change in the carrying angle of the neck, painful walking, and less ability to exercise. Over 250,000 women each year have hip fractures and 15% of these die within 4 months of the fracture; caring for these patients costs an estimated 5-7 billion dollars yearly.

Since mass screening for osteoporosis is impractical and cannot identify at age 40 years those women at risk for fracture 30 years later, identification of risk factors for the development of osteoporosis is important and helpful. Women who are at greater risk for the development of osteoporosis can be identified. By the time the diagnosis of osteoporosis is made, either by dual photon absorptiometry, or CT scanning, years of prevention have already been lost.

Risk Factors for the Development of Osteoporosis

Family history of osteoporosis	Nulliparity
Thin body habitus	Gastric or small-bowel resection
Sedentary, nonexercising	Long-term glucocorticoid therapy
Poor nutritional habits	Long-term use of anti-convulsants
Poor calcium intake	Hyperparathyroidism
Caucasian	Thyrotoxicosis
Premature menopause	Smoking
Short stature and small bones	Heavy alcohol use

There are two types of osteoporosis, type I, which is estrogen-associated, and type II, which is calcium-associated.

Type I: Predominantly affects trabecular bone in women more so than men, accelerates shortly after menopause, and is related to estrogen deprivation. Bones predominantly affected are the vertebra (crush fractures) and the distal radius. Parathyroid function is decreased, calcium absorption decreased, and there is a secondary decrease in metabolism of 25-OH vitamin D to 1,25 (OH)$_2$ vitamin D. Type I osteoporosis is primarily prevented by estrogen replacement.

Type II: Affects both trabecular and cortical bone in both men and women, and occurs after age 70 years. Bones affected include the vertebra and the hip. Parathyroid function is increased, calcium absorption decreased, and there is a primary decrease of metabolism of 25-OH-vitamin D to 1,25 dihydroxyvitamin D. Type II osteoporosis responds quite satisfactorily to a regimen of calcium and exercise, particularly as prevention.

Prophylaxis for osteoporosis should begin at or before age 35 years, with calcium supplementation 600 mg daily combined with 45 minutes daily walking or weight-bearing forms of exercise. Since 50% of the bone mass which will be lost occurs in the 7 years after menopause, estrogen replacement is indicated as prophylaxis, perhaps in all women who have no contraindication.

The mechanism of action of estrogen may be indirect, as bone lacks estrogen receptors. Urinary calcium and hydroxyproline are reduced; in estrogen-treated patients, urinary cyclic AMP is increased; osteoclast function is reduced; calcium absorption from the gut is increased; renal production of 1,25 dihydroxyvitamin D is increased; serum PTH is increased; and serum phosphate and serum calcium are decreased.

Either there is increased anabolic activity of parathyroid hormone (PTH) or an increased skeletal resistance to the catabolic effects of PTH. Estrogen also stimulates calcitonin production, which prevents bone loss. Decreased bone resorption leads to reduced serum calcium which stimulates plasma thromboplastin antecedent (PTA) production which stimulates renal hydroxylation of 25-hydroxyvitamin D to 1,25 dihydroxyvitamin D which stimulates calcium absorption from the gastrointestinal tract which reduces bone turnover further; increased PTH changes phosphate metabolism and decreased urinary hydroxyprolene output occurs directly from inhibition of osteoclast activity.

EXPECTED RESULTS FROM ESTROGEN REPLACEMENT THERAPY (ERT)

THE BENEFITS OF ERT

1. Suppression of vasomotor symptoms
2. Reversed atrophy of the genitourinary system
3. Retardation and prevention of osteoporosis
4. Increased quality of life
5. Psychologic benefits due to improved REM sleep (no waking due to a hot flash) with decreased tiredness, fatigue, irritability, and confusion
6. Probable prevention of atheroscerotic heart disease
7. Other beneficial effects including dermatologic, sexual, and attitudinal benefits

THE RISK:BENEFIT RATIO WITH ERT

The benefits versus the risks of hormone replacement therapy must be carefully considered for each patient. In certain circumstances, risks clearly outweigh the benefits, and estrogen replacement therapy is contraindicated.

ABSOLUTE CONTRAINDICATIONS TO ERT

1. Breast cancer
2. Endometrial cancer
3. Impaired liver function
4. Gall bladder disease
5. Acute liver disease
6. Thromboembolism
7. Severe thrombophlebitis
8. Unexplained vaginal bleeding
9. Acute vascular thrombosis

RELATIVE CONTRAINDICATIONS
WEIGHED ACCORDING TO THEIR IMPORTANCE
REQUIRE CLOSE MONITORING

1. Hypertension
2. Uterine fibroid tumors
3. Seizure disorders
4. Familial hyperlipidemia
5. Migraine headaches
6. History of liver disease
7. Endometriosis
8. Family history of estrogen-dependent neoplasia
9. Diabetes mellitus
10. Porphyria
11. Ischemic heart disease

RISKS AND COMPLICATIONS OF ERT

Neoplasia

Endometrial Cancer: Unopposed ERT predisposes to the
development of endometrial hyperplasia and to carcinoma.
Postmenopausal women who use no hormone therapy have an incidence of
endometrial cancer of about 245/100,000; a 60% increase in incidence
is associated with estrogen treatment alone and cyclic use of
estrogen alone does not protect against cancer. The cancer is only
minimally invasive and has a 95% 5-year survival. However, the risk
is significantly lower (49/100,000) in women treated with an
estrogen plus progestin combination regimen, and few if any cases of
carcinoma have been reported in patients receiving 10 days of
progestin each cycle.

Breast Cancer: Estrogen or progestin alone may reduce the
incidence of breast cancer from 350 to 150/100,000 whereas estrogen
plus progestin is associated with a significant reduction in the
incidence to 68/100,000. A protective effect against the
development of breast cancer has been postulated; the incidence of
breast cancer has not paralleled the use of estrogen in the U.S.
Estrogen can induce cystic and/or dysplastic breast changes. Some
breast cancers are estrogen dependent, so the presence of breast
cancer is a contraindication to the use of estrogen replacement
therapy.

Liver: Estrogens are metabolized in the first pass through the
hepatocytes after gastrointestinal absorption, so the hepatic
effects of estrogen are significant. Hepatic synthesis of
angiotensinogen, the renin substrate, is stimulated; thromboembolic
phenomena are not increased by replacement doses of estrogen, but

there is at least a minimal effect on hepatic clotting factor synthesis. The increased incidence of gallbladder problems is probably due to the estrogen induced increase in cholesterol saturation of the bile.

Cardiovascular Disease

There is probably a relationship between estrogen deprivation and the development of heart disease. The protective effect of low-dose estrogen is mediated through a decrease in low-density lipoproteins (LDL) and an increase in high-density lipoproteins (HDL). Both systolic and diastolic blood pressures may be decreased by estrogen replacement. There is now general agreement that estrogen treatment does not increase the risk of arteriosclerotic cardiovascular disease (ASCVD) and may be protective.

MANAGEMENT REGIMENS

There are many forms of estrogen clinically available. The most commonly used are conjugated estrogens, composed of over 8 various forms of estrogen, but predominating in estrone and estrone sulfate. Micronized 17β-estradiol (estrace) is absorbed orally, with a good record of efficacy. Estriols were proposed as being less biologically active, and thereby less apt to induce endometrial hyperplasia; this theory has not worked out in practice.

```
Available estrogens
    1) conjugated steroidal estrogens
            Estrones:       Conjugated equine estrogens
                            Esterified estrogens
                            Piperazine estrone sulfate
            Estradiols:     Estradiol cypionate
                            Estradiol valerate
                            Micronized 17β-estradiol
            Estriols:       Estriol
                            Estriol hemisuccinate
    2) nonconjugated steroidal estrogens
            17-ethinyl estradiol
            17-ethinyl estradiol-3-methyl-ether (mestranol)
            17-ethinyl-estradiol-3-cyclopentoether (quinestrol)
    3) synthetic estrogen analogues (nonsteroids)
            Stilbene derivatives (e.g., DES)
            Naphthalene derivatives
```

BIOLOGIC POTENCY

17β-estradiol is the most potent of the three main estrogens due to its long half-life. Estriol is rapidly and readily oxidized to estrone, and estradiol reaches the systemic circulation in this form when administered orally. Estrone has a half-life of approximately 24 hours, and is of intermediate potency. Estriol is considered a short-acting estrogen with a half-life of 5 hours.

	Vaginal Cornification	Antigonadotropin	Anti-Implantation
Estradiol	100	100	100
Estrone	30	30	70
Estriol	3	10	12
Ethinyl estradiol	150	300	70
Mestranol	10	100	20

The oral administration of micronized estradiol results in a four-fold rise in serum estradiol and a 20-fold increase in serum estrone after 4-6 hours. Estrone sulfate is also a product of the conversion of estradiol to estrone, and there is little transfer back from either of the estrones to estradiol. Estrone sulfate has a metabolic clearance rate 1/12 that of estrone, converts readily back to estrone, has a large volume of distribution, and can become a pool for regeneration of free steroid. Estrone and estrone sulfate are excreted in the urine in the forms of glucuronides and sulfates; estrone sulfate is excreted as such in the urine, and estrone is converted to estrone glucuronide.

Administration of conjugated equine estrogens, consisting of 50% estrone sulfate and 25% equilin sulfate as the major constituents, results in high equilin levels which, due to a reduced metabolic clearance can be measured in the blood of women 3 months following therapy with conjugated estrogens.

The administration of synthetic estrogens, including ethinyl estradiol, mestranol and quinestrol, results in less gut or liver metabolism than 17β-estradiol, although the first-pass effect is still approximately 50%. Mestranol is rapidly metabolized to ethinyl estradiol, and 30-45% of the oral ethinyl estradiol dose is excreted in the urine over 8 days, suggesting that there is a large pool in the body that is only slowly excreted.

The routes of administration may be:
  (1) oral
  (2) vaginal
  (3) implant
  (4) transdermal
  (5) other

The route of administration determines the circulating product. Oral administration of micronized 17β-estradiol results in a rapid metabolic conversion to estrone which takes place primarily in the liver and gastrointestinal tract, causing a potent biologic effect. Sublingual administration results in a dramatic increase in serum estradiol, 3.5 times greater than the increase in serum estrone. The conversion to estrone by the sublingual compared to the oral route is similar, but with a delayed peak of estrone.

Vaginal administration of micronized 17β-estradiol results in rapid absorption with an immediate increase in the E_2-to-estrone ratio, and a slower conversion to estrone. The advantage of the vaginal route is a decreased first-pass effect on the liver. Vaginal administration of conjugated estrogens exerts mainly a local effect, with limited changes in systemic markers. Both oral and vaginal routes of administration result in relief of vasomotor symptomatology, but each is associated with development of endometrial hyperplasia if progestin is not added. The major difference between the two routes is how they affect hepatic metabolism, specifically the synthesis of plasma proteins and globulins, clotting factors and lipoproteins.

Transdermal and subcutaneous implants of estradiol result in an elevated E_2-to-estrone ratio, and with a high bioavailability of estrogens to target organs.

Administration Regimens

Various cyclic estrogen administration regimens have been used, most commonly on days 1-25 of the month. Recent information suggests that continuous administration might result in less endometrial stimulation than with cyclic therapy. The incidence of hyperplasia with continuous therapy was 3.7/100 women-months, and with cyclic administration was 4.5/100 women-months, not a significant difference.

PROGESTINS

The addition of progestin to therapy is protective to the endometrium, and may be administered in either a cyclic or a continuous fashion. Studies indicate that at least 12 and better 14 days of progestin administration is necessary in any monthly cycle.

Progestin administration is essential in women with an intact uterus, and perhaps for protection of the breast. Available progestins include: norethindrone, 1-10 mg daily; norgestrel, 150-500 µg daily; medroxyprogesterone acetate 10 mg daily; and progesterone, 300 mg daily.

Progestins may be additive in the beneficial effect of estrogen in the prevention of osteoporosis. The minimum effective dose of estrogen for prevention of postmenopausal bone loss is 0.625 mg conjugated estrogen. If micronized 17β-estradiol is used, 1 mg of orally administered 17β-estradiol daily in a 21-day cyclic regimen is as effective as 0.625 conjugated estrogens.

EXERCISE

Exercise, particularly weight bearing, is essential in the prophylaxis and prevention of osteoporosis. At least 45 minutes a day of fast walking is beneficial.

CALCIUM SUPPLEMENTATION

Dietary calcium intake is below the requirement necessary for maintenance of bone. Women over the age of 35 years may supplement with about 600 mg calcium daily, and postmenopausal women should supplement with 1200 mg calcium daily. Calcium supplements available vary considerably, with calcium citrate being the best absorbed. Patients complain of bloating, and other gastrointestinal problems. A dose of 1 g elemental calcium daily in addition to normal dietary intake is needed to meet postmenopausal requirements.

FLUORIDE

Fluoride increases bone formation with an increase in trabecular bone mass. Fluoride, however, impairs mineralization of the increased osteoid tissue, suggestive of osteomalacia and producing brittle bones; this can be helped, but not totally prevented by calcium supplementation. Cortical bone mass is lost during fluoride administration, and there may be an increased risk of fracture of the proximal femur in fluoride-treated patients. There is a high incidence of rheumatic and gastrointestinal symptoms.

VITAMIN D

Vitamin D, or the more potent analogues 1-α, 25 dihydroxy-vitamin D_3 (calcitriol) and 1-α-hydroxy-vitamin D_3 (α-calcidol) lead to an increased absorption of calcium from the gut. However, vitamin D administration alone cannot increase calcium balance sufficiently, and there is no increase in bone mineral content. Vitamin D administration is not an essential part of the therapy of osteoporosis.

CALCITONIN

Calcitonin inhibits bone resorption, and is probably effective in treating osteoporosis. Salmon calcitonin produces a temporary increase in total body calcium by decreasing bone resorption. The major complication is flushing after the injection; the problems of expense and inconvenience of parental administration make calcitonin an unusually chosen form of therapy.

ANABOLIC STEROIDS

Stanozolol is an anabolic steroid which increases total body calcium in postmenopausal osteoporotic women. Side-effects are common, and in one study, the vertebral fracture rate was not significantly reduced. This therapy cannot presently be recommended for general use.

OVERALL RECOMMENDATIONS FOR THERAPY

1. Estrogen should be used for an indication, in the smallest effective dose and for the shortest time period that satisfies therapeutic need. In the situation of osteoporosis, this may be life-time.
2. Estrogens are effective in the treatment of prevention of vasomotor flushes, atrophic urogenital conditions, and osteoporosis.
3. Estrogens may have a protective effect against certain manifestations of arteriosclerotic heart disease.
4. When estrogen is given to menopausal women with intact uteri, progestin administration must be added. There is some evidence that continuous versus cyclic estrogen therapy is beneficial. There is evidence that at least 10 days and perhaps more of progestin administration is needed.
5. Topical estrogen preparations are useful in the treatment of vulvo-vaginal atrophic problems. Absorption is rapid and if there are contraindications to the administration of estrogen orally, then these contraindications are not bypassed by vaginal administration.
6. Any vaginal bleeding must be investigated promptly.
7. Yearly monitoring of asymptomatic patients is necessary, including histologic or cytologic sampling of the endometrium, pelvic and breast examinations. Blood pressure should be measured, and mammography accomplished.
8. Estrogen replacement therapy is specifically contraindicated in patients with an estrogen-dependent neoplasm.

SUGGESTED READING

Brenner PF: Estrogen replacement therapy: An overview. Int J Fertil 31:7, 1986.

Cummings SR, Black D: Should perimenopausal women be screened for osteoporosis? Ann Intern Med 104:817, 1986.

Ettinger B, Genant HK, Cann CE: Long-term estrogen replacement prevents bone loss and fractures. Ann Intern Med 102:319, 1985.

Gambrell RD Jr: Cancer and the use of estrogens. Int J Fertil 31:112, 1986.

Judd HL, Shamonki IM, Frumar AM, Lagasse LD: Origin of serum estradiol in postmenopausal women. Obstet Gynecol 59:680, 1982.

Nichols KC, Schenkel L, Benson H: 17β-estradiol for postmenopausal estrogen replacement therapy. Obstet Gynecol Surv 39:230, 1984.

Upton GV: The contraceptive and hormonal requirements of the premenopausal woman: The years from forty to fifty. Int J Fertil 30:44, 1986.

Whitehead M, Lane G, Siddle N, Townsend P, King R: Avoidance of endometrial hyperstimulation in estrogen-treated postmenopausal women. Sem Reproduc Endocrinol 1:41, 1983.

Woolf AD, Dixon ASJ: Osteoporosis. An update on management. Drugs 28:565, 1984.

Office of Medical Applications of Research of NIH: Osteoporosis. JAMA 252:799, 1984.

Chapter 11

Overview of Infertility

Anne Colston Wentz, M.D.

INTRODUCTION

Involuntary sterility affects an estimated 15% of couples or about one in every seven marriages. In the 1980's, there are more infertile couples than ever before who have delayed their child-bearing for career and other reasons and who want their child-bearing condensed into a shorter period of time. An increasing proportion of these couples are seeking care, with high expectation of a solution. There is a greater demand for physicians to deal with infertility and more sophisticated methods of diagnosis and approaches to treatment.

DEFINITIONS

Fecundity: the physical ability of a woman or couple to conceive and/or to have children.

Sterility: absolute total inability to have children.

Infertility: a medical concept which identifies couples that may need medical services to improve their chances of becoming pregnant.

Primary infertility: involuntary failure to achieve pregnancy, where the female partner has not previously been pregnant.

Secondary infertility: involuntary infertility with proven past fertility, including ectopic gestations. Recurrent early pregnancy wastage is considered a form of secondary infertility.

EVALUATING INFERTILITY: GENERALITIES

Patients in the reproductive age group, who have not achieved pregnancy with at least 1 year of exposure, deserve an evaluation. Certain individuals in our society feel that proof of fertility is essential before marriage, and these cases are to be handled individually. Others have some reason to suspect infertility (pelvic inflammatory disease, varicocele) and their evaluation might be undertaken if they present before a year of unprotected intercourse.

Ideally, both husband and wife should participate together in the evaluation. It is appropriate to interview each alone, beginning with the wife, and talking with the husband while she is readied for her examination. The husband should be with the wife during her physical and pelvic examination, and for the consultation which follows. According to practicality, the husband and wife should be together for all subsequent testing.

From the initial encounter, openness and a willingness to answer questions is important. The basic infertility evaluation should be completely and thoroughly explained. Handouts and booklets describing the procedures are helpful. Alternatives must be mentioned. An infertility evaluation must be considered to be entirely elective. Since office visits and diagnostic tests may not be covered by insurance, it is helpful to explain to a couple what their financial responsibilities are likely to be, and what demands will be made on their time.

GOALS

The goals of an infertility evaluation are two-fold:
(1) to discover the etiology of past infertility
(2) to provide a prognosis for future fertility

Pregnancy in all cases is an unreasonable goal both for patient and physician. Some patients will decide to terminate the evaluation when a diagnosis has been obtained, others will elect to pursue adoption, and some will continue with the medical or surgical therapy advised. For a statistical appreciation of the overall results to be expected from an infertility evaluation, it is just as important to know the number who elected not to proceed with therapy.

142

THE BASIC INFERTILITY EVALUATION

The infertility investigation considers three areas:

(1) age of the wife
(2) duration of the history
(3) the factor responsible

The age of maximal fertility in the female is approximately 24 years, and the maximum age for a successful pregnancy in women is about 52 years old. At age 25 years, 74.6% of conceptions occur in less than 6 months; between ages 35 and 39 years, only 25.5% occur in less than 6 months; and after age 40 years, the number drops to 22.7%. Fecundity appears to be decreasing in the female at the age of 30 years, but a significant difference cannot be found until after the age of 35 years. From the psychological and physiological standpoint, it seems important to institute an infertility evaluation without delay after age 30 years.

Approximately 60-70% of couples will achieve pregnancy within 6 months, 80% in 9 months, and 90% within 1 year. A couple having unprotected intercourse for at least a year is considered to be infertile and unlikely to achieve pregnancy without medical evaluation. The duration of exposure to pregnancy helps to determine the prognosis for future fertility; the longer the couple have been married without achieving pregnancy, the greater the progressive decline in conception rate.

The third major area to be considered is the medical factor responsible for the infertility. The six medical factors which must be evaluated are:

(1) Central or ovulatory factor
(2) Male factor
(3) Mucus or cervical factor
(4) Endometrial-uterine factor
(5) Tubal factor
(6) Peritoneal or pelvic factor

A seventh area, the psychogenic factor, may also play a role.

Having explored the basics by history and examination, a definite plan, with a predictable end point, should be established for the couple. A routine screening infertility evaluation should be almost complete in three office visits. Five of the six infertility factors can be evaluated in one ovulatory cycle. Since two or more factors have been found to be operative in fully 35% of all infertility cases, it is essential that both partners be thoroughly evaluated. If all factors have been investigated completely, a diagnosis to explain the infertility will be found in about 95% of couples.

BEGINNING THE WORK-UP

1. Take a thorough history. A complete and detailed history, and competent physical examination must be performed on every patient. The history must completely elucidate any and all factors which could be responsible for infertility. A thorough family history, past medical history, sexual and social history are essential. Results of previous evaluations and treatment must be obtained from other physicians. Operative notes and discharge summaries are essential. Actual x-rays and slides of biopsy material should be reviewed.

2. Do a thorough examination. A complete physical examination details abnormalities found in systems other than the reproductive. Note pattern of hair growth, signs of weight gain or loss, skin color, abdominal incisional scars, and striae. Look for anomalies of the cervix, uterus, or vagina. (Evaluate the quantity and quality of cervical mucus and search for evidence of cervical cautery, cryosurgery, conization, or stigmata of DES exposure.) Examine uterine contour, shape, and mobility.

3. Put the patient on a basal temperature chart. The basal body temperature chart is the simplest and cheapest presumptive means of determining (in retrospect) that ovulation has occurred. It is used by the physician to schedule and interpret tests used in the infertility evaluation.

Technique:

1. The patient is instructed in reading a thermometer.
2. The first day of menses is considered day 1 of the cycle, and a new chart is begun with the onset of menses.
3. The thermometer is shaken down and placed within reach the night before.
4. The oral temperature should be taken in bed at the same time every morning, weekends and holidays included, before any activity, such as toothbrushing, eating or smoking. The temperature may be written down later in the day.
5. Intercourse, illnesses, spotting, vaginal discharge, or dysmenorrheic pain should be recorded on the chart.
6. The chart is not to be used to time intercourse, or for the patient to interpret her own cycle.
7. The temperature chart must be brought to every office visit.

Interpretation: In the proliferative part of the cycle, or in any anovulatory cycle, the oral temperature is usually in the low 97s. About the time of ovulation, some charts will show a slight

144

drop in temperature, prior to what is called the continuous rise. The temperature will rise at least 0.6-0.8°F and will be in the 98s. The duration of the luteal phase is timed from the lowest point before the continuous rise to the onset of menses. The luteal phase should last 14 + 2 days. Ovulation probably occurs during the 48 hours prior to the continuous rise but this is impossible to predict exactly.

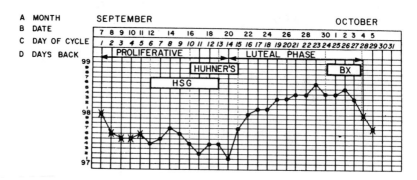

The Basal Body Temperature Chart. The postcoital test (Huhner's or PCT) is properly performed during the 3 days before the temperature rise. The endometrial biopsy (Bx) should be taken within 1-2 days of the expected menses. The hysterosalpingogram (HSG) is performed when menstrual bleeding has ceased and before ovulation occurs, and can be done the same day as the PCT. The semen analysis can be done the same day as the biopsy. Five of the six infertility factors can be evaluated in one ovulatory cycle.

The basal temperature chart cannot establish that ovulation is occurring, but it can aid in the scheduling and interpretation of tests. Follicular shortening, late ovulation, luteal shortening, and delayed menses are easily observed. Proper timing for postcoital tests and endometrial biopsies can be decided and pregnancy diagnosed early. If the temperature chart is used for scheduling and interpretation, and not to time intercourse, the anxiety-provoking aspects are greatly lessened.

The patient should be asked to record daily temperatures only for the limited time necessary to complete the basic infertility evaluation. The woman who is no longer actively undergoing

infertility testing can take her basal temperature for 7-10 days
each cycle and produce useful information; this includes the date of
last period, subsequent period, and when the chart became biphasic.
Have the regularly cycling woman begin temperature taking about
cycle day 12 and stop when the temperature has clearly risen.

For women who work nights and sleep days, the temperature chart
can still be valuable: simply have her take her temperature when she
is basal, after 3 or 4 hours of uninterrupted sleep.

All happenings of interest should be recorded on the chart,
including late nights, alcohol consumption, sickness, intercourse,
bleeding, cramping or spotting, and so forth. Importantly, the
keeping of a temperature chart should not be open-ended, and the
chart itself should only be used for scheduling and interpretation
of tests.

   4. Schedule the Basic Infertility Evaluation. The etiologic
cause is sought by performing specific tests and procedures. The
PCT and HSG should be scheduled in the late proliferative phase just
before ovulation; and the sperm count and endometrial biopsy in the
late luteal phase, just before menstruation.

FACTOR	PROCEDURE
A. Central or ovulatory factor	History, basal temperature chart
B. Male factor	Semen analysis, examination by urologist
C. Cervical or mucus factor	PCT; sperm-mucus penetration tests
D. Endometrial or uterine factor	Timed, dated endometrial biopsy;
E. Tubal factor	Hysterosalpingography; methylene blue or indigo carmine dye injection at laparoscopy
F. Peritoneal factor	Diagnostic laparoscopy
G. Psychogenic factor	History

UNEXPLAINED INFERTILITY

Finally, what can one expect in the couple in whom a thorough infertility evaluation has been completed, without finding the etiologic reason for the infertility? Recent studies suggest that only 3.5% of couples fail to show some etiologic factor associated with infertility; the 10-20% incidence of unexplained infertility quoted earlier is too high an estimate in view of the additional information made available through pelvic endoscopy. However, the so-called "normal infertile couple" is a misnomer; these patients are obviously not normal. However, this factor offers a good prognosis, as 60% of couples with no identified factor will achieve pregnancy within 3 years of completing the evaluation. On the other hand, a couple who has not become pregnant within 36 months is <u>very</u> unlikely to do so later.

CONCLUSION

Most success in the management of infertility is achieved if an etiologic reason for the infertility is found. If therapy is based upon the discovered etiology, a prognosis for future fertility can be made for the couple. With incidence of the normal infertile couple will be decreased, and the goals of an infertility evaluation will have been accomplished.

SUGGESTED READING

Aral SO, Cates W Jr: The increasing concern with infertility. JAMA 250:2327, 1983.

Collins JA, Wrixon W, Janes LB, Wilson EH: Treatment-independent pregnancy among infertile couples. N Engl J Med 309:1201, 1983.

Jones WR: Immunologic infertility - fact or fiction? Fertil Steril 33:577, 1980.

Leridon H, Spira A: Problems in measuring the effectiveness of infertility therapy. Fertil Steril 41:580, 1984.

Steinberger E, Rodriguez-Rigau LJ: The infertile couple. J Androl 4:111, 1983.

Verkauf BS: The incidence and outcome of single-factor, multifactorial, and unexplained infertility. Am J Obstet Gynecol 147:175, 1983.

Chapter 12

The Ovulatory Factor and Ovulation Inducement

George A. Hill, M.D.

INTRODUCTION

Ovulatory dysfunction is present in approximately 15-25% of couples presenting for an infertility evaluation. Proper diagnosis with appropriate selection of therapy is essential in order to maximize the pregnancy rate and minimize complications.

CAUSES OF ANOVULATION (Since anovulation is frequently associated with amenorrhea, refer to Chapter 3 for further information regarding differential diagnosis, evaluation, and therapy)

PRETREATMENT EVALUATION

1. Document oligo or anovulation by history, basal body temperature chart, or serum progesterone.
2. Evaluate the endometrium to exclude endometrial hyperplasia in the amenorrheic, hyperestrogenic patient.
3. Exclude hyperprolactinemia, thyroid or adrenal dysfunction, hepatic disorders, and pregnancy.
4. Exclude ovarian failure.
5. Evaluate other infertility factors (male, tubal, peritoneal, cervical).
6. Obtain informed consent from the patient. Review the costs, risks to the mother and fetus, chance of multiple births, side effects, complications, abortion rates, success rates, and alternative forms of therapy.

SELECTION OF PATIENTS

In general, patients with anovulation presenting for ovulation induction may be classified into three groups:

148

Group I: Hypogonadotrophic, Hypoestrogenic

This group consists of patients with amenorrhea, who are hypoestrogenic, and who may have a history of postpill amenorrhea, severe mental distress, or marked weight loss, or who are known to have hypogonadotropic ovarian failure, partial or complete hypopituitarism, or aquired pituitary-hypothalamic dysfunction. Patients with either primary or secondary amenorrhea may fit this classification.

Physical examination reveals evidence of a low estrogen milieu, with small breasts or a decrease in breast size, an atrophic vaginal mucosa, and a poor or absent cervical mucus. The endometrial biopsy will be atrophic or proliferative, and ordinarily is an unnecessary procedure in hypoestrogenic women. Serum gonadotropin levels may be low or low-normal. Progesterone withdrawal usually does not induce menstrual bleeding, as predicted from the hypoestrogenic vaginal examination, and is also unnecessary.

The treatment of choice in these patients is usually human menopausal gonadotropin (hMG) (Pergonal) plus human chorionic gonadotropin (hCG), although a trial of clomiphene citrate (CC) is first indicated. These patients should theoretically respond to luteinizing hormone releasing hormone (GnRH). However, an isolated pituitary gonadotroph defect must first be excluded by appropriate stimulatory tests with GnRH.

Group II: Normogonadotropic, Normoestrogenic

These are patients with anovulation or oligo-ovulation, who have evidence of endogenous estrogen activity, and a distinctive gonadotropin pattern revealing an elevated luteinizing hormone (LH) and normal or low follicle stimulating hormone (FSH) output. A history of obesity, hirsutism, acne, or dysfunctional bleeding may be obtained, or the patient may have previously been diagnosed to have polycystic ovarian disease or rarely, postpubertal adrenal hyperplasia.

Physical examination reveals an increased estrogen milieu, frequently associated with stigmata of excess androgen production. The vaginal mucosa has an abundance of cornified cells, the cervical mucus is lush, and the endometrium may reveal a benign hyperplasia, or atypical changes.

In these patients, clomiphene induction of ovulation is the treatment of choice, once the endometrial pattern has been established. Ordinarily, ovulation induction is simple; however, some of these women are brittle, may hyperstimulate on low doses of CC, or may be resistant to CC. Some may have failure of the LH surge, and the addition of hCG may be necessary.

Group III: Hypergonadotropic, Hypoestrogenic

These are patients with amenorrhea, who are hypoestrogenic and may have a history of hot flashes or other vasomotor complaints. These patients are differentiated from those in Group I by their markedly elevated serum gonadotropins, and have ovarian failure or premature menopause.

Recently, several patients have been reported with secondary amenorrhea and massively elevated gonadotropin, who have had ovarian biopsy evidence of persistent primordial follicles. Comparison has been made to the "insensitive ovary syndrome" in which primary amenorrhea is associated with the above findings and which is thought to be due to an FSH membrane receptor defect. Although ovulation induction has been stimulated in some with hugh Pergonal doses, pregnancy has not been documented. Thus, there is little justification to treat these patients with Pergonal and no reason to recommend that an ovarian biopsy be obtained in the patient who presents with massively elevated gonadotropins.

TREATMENT

1. CLOMIPHENE CITRATE

CC is a triphenylethylene derivative with weak estrogenic and strong antiestrogenic effects. It possesses no progestational, corticotropic, androgenic, or antiandrogenic properties and initiates ovulation via its actions at the level of the hypothalamus, the pituitary, and possibly the ovary. CC has an estimated half-life of approximately 5 days in the human.
   A. The hypothalamic effects are mainly antiestrogenic.

> The ability of CC to initiate ovulation is due primarily to its ability to be recognized by and interact with estrogen receptors at the level of the hypothalamus.
>
> CC is thought to displace endogenous estrogen from hypothalamic estrogen receptor sites, thereby alleviating the negative feedback effect exerted by endogenous estrogens.
>
> CC has been shown to cause an increase in the pulse frequency of LH and FSH with little or no effect on the pulse amplitude, giving

indirect evidence that the primary mode of
action of CC is at the level of the
hypothalamus.

B. The pituitary effects appear to be primarily
estrogenic.

CC may exert a direct stimulatory effect on
gonadotropin release by the pituitary,
independent of its ability to alter the
pattern of GnRH release.

This direct estrogenic action may consist in
part of sensitization of the gonadotrope to
the action of GnRH.

C. The ovarian effects appear to be estrogenic.

CC may act directly at the ovary or may
synergize with pituitary gonadotropins in this
connection.

D. Cervical effects appear to be antiestrogenic.

CC will antagonize the effects of exogenously
administered ethinyl estradiol on vaginal
cytology, cervical mucus, and uterine
morphology of ovariectomized women.

CC will decrease the quantity and quality of
cervical mucus in ovulatory women receiving CC,
150 mg for five days, despite increased levels
of serum estradiol.

The summation of these effects produces an increase in both FSH
and LH to initiate follicular development.

Hormonal Response Expected

If serial gonadotropin values are measured during CC
administration, one observes an immediate increase in FSH, which
usually drops by day 4 or 5 of CC administration. The increase in
LH begins somewhat more slowly and continues throughout the entire
course of CC, decreasing a day or two after discontinuation. Thus,
one can change the dosage or duration to effect an appropriate
hormonal response in properly selected patients. In the patient
suspected to have a poor FSH stimulation, an increase in dosage in
the next cycle is indicated. On the other hand, if a failure of LH

output is suspected, reflected by a poor estrogenic response, then a longer duration of CC administration may be effective. If ovulation does not occur, but an excellent estrogenic mucus is observed some 12-14 days after beginning CC, then HCG 5000-10,000 I.U. should be added to substitute for the LH surge, and to act as a luteotropic agent.

Expected Results

A 50-70% ovulation rate may be expected with CC administration, but pregnancy figures are usually 40% or less. The multiple pregnancy rate is approximately 6-10%; and fetal wastage, mostly early miscarriage, occurs in 25-35% of pregnancies,compared to a miscarriage rate of 15-20% in the general population.

The discrepancy between ovulation and pregnancy rates has several explanations:

1. About one-third of patients undergoing ovulation induction with CC may have luteal phase inadequacy as diagnosed by the timed, dated endometrial biopsy. The luteal phase inadequacy can result in frank infertility, occult miscarriage, or early miscarriage. Thus, the adequacy of corpus luteum function must be ascertained in the first ovulatory CC cycle. Treatment of the luteal phase inadequacy is relatively simple, and results in an increased pregnancy rate and decreased miscarriage rate if begun before the first missed menses.

2. An ovulatory response may be difficult to diagnose unless serial progesterone levels or the endometrial biopsy is utilized, so the ovulation rate may be falsely elevated.

3. CC may be retained in the estrogen receptor sites of the endocervical glands for a longer period of time, resulting in a poor mucus response unfavorable for sperm penetration.

4. In the general population, 60% of couples achieve pregnancy within 6 months; the number of CC courses administered may have been inadequate to have achieved a reasonable rate of pregnancy.

The incidence of adverse outcome in pregnancies (as measured by abortion, stillbirth, or birth anomalies) associated with the use of CC remains within the expected range of the general United States population. In an analysis of 2369 pregnancies, 58 infants (2.5%)

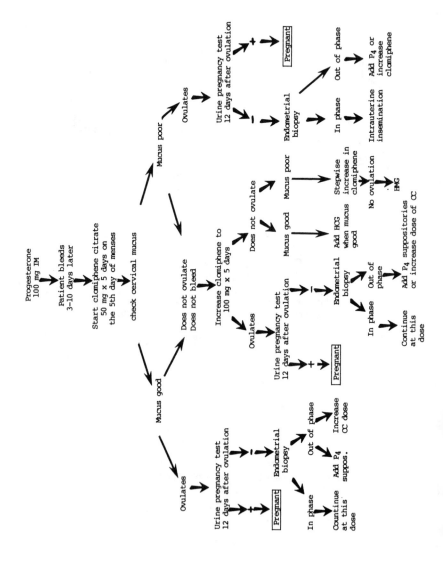

were born with birth anomalies. In a study of 158 mothers who took CC during pregnancy, 8 infants (5.0%) were born with birth anomalies. These numbers fall within the expected range of the normal population.

Techniques of Monitoring

In the first CC cycle, it is important to document an estrogenic mucus response and the normality of corpus luteum function. A temperature chart should be maintained to aid in interpretation and scheduling of tests. CC may be begun on the third or fifth day of bleeding, either spontaneous or induced by progesterone. This serves as a marker for the patient for subsequent courses and assurance that the patient is not pregnant. Most patients receiving CC for 5 days will ovulate 12-16 days after beginning CC. The presence and adequacy of cervical mucus should be documented 12-14 days into the CC cycle. In the infertile patient, this is an ideal time for a postcoital test (PCT). Most patients with an adequate estrogen milieu will ovulate, and menstruate 12-14 days later. The patient, therefore, should be seen just before the expected menses for an endometrial biopsy to document the endometrial response to progesterone output from the corpus luteum. If an inadequate luteal phase is diagnosed, therapy may be instituted in the form of either progesterone vaginal suppositories or the addition of HCG in subsequent cycles. It is not useful to increase the dose of CC under these circumstances.

If the patient fails to ovulate in the first CC course, there is no advantage to administering a similar clomiphene dose in the next cycle. Most conveniently, if the patient has failed to ovulate on 50 mg for 5 days, the dose is increased to 100 mg for 5 days. If an excellent cervical mucus response is observed in the second cycle, and the patient does not ovulate, hCG 10,000 I.U. may be added in the next cycle. Increasing the CC dose is not helpful as hyperstimulated ovaries are likely and the good mucus suggests that FSH stimulation has been adequate; what is lacking is the LH surge, which can be substituted for with HCG. The importance of monitoring the patient's estrogenic response is therefore emphasized.

The figure on the preceding page provides a guide for the use of CC in ovulation induction.

Adverse Effects

Hot Flashes: May occur in up to 11% of patients. The mechanism of action is thought to be an apparent state of estrogen deprivation consequent to CC effecting an estrogen receptor blockade.

Multiple Gestation: This is due almost exclusively to multiple ovlation resulting from the higher levels of gonadotropins induced in CC initiated ovulatory cycles. A large study revealed an overall figure of 7.9%, of which 6.9% were twins, 0.5% were triplets, 0.3% quadruplets, and 0.13% quintuplets.

Visual Symptoms: These occur in less that 2% of patients treated with CC. They are generally described as "blurring" or spots or flashes (scintillatory scotomota) and have been correlated with increasing total dose. These symptoms tend to disappear within a few days after CC is discontinued. Patients having any visual symptoms should discontinue treatment and consideration should be given to other modes of ovulation initiation.

2. GLUCOCORTICOIDS

Adrenal androgen production reflected by an increase in the serum dehydroepiandrosterone sulfate (DS) or urinary 17-ketosteroids may block ovulation attempts with CC. In patients with a serum DS >200 µg %, the addition of dexamethasone resulted in a significantly higher rate of ovulation and conception. There was no advantage of adding dexamethasone in the anovulatory patient whose serum DS was <200 µg %. Therefore, patients with elevated serum DS levels who fail to ovulate on normal doses of CC may benefit by the addition of dexamethasone, 0.25 or 0.5 mg daily at night, to suppress the adrenal contribution to the androgen pool.

3. HUMAN MENOPAUSAL GONADOTROPINS (HMG) (PERGONAL)

Mechanism

HMG (Pergonal) contains 75 I.U.s of FSH and 75 I.U.s of LH in each ampule. These purified gonadotropins, derived from the urine of menopausal women, directly stimulate ovarian folliculogenesis.

Indications

1. In the hypoestrogenic patient who does not respond to maximum doses of CC, HMG may be utilized (although GnRH may also work well - see next section).

2. HMG is the drug of choice in patients who have pituitary disorders as the cause of their anovulation.

3. HMG may also be useful in the patient who ovulates on CC,
   but has a poor cervical mucus response. If all other
   modalities to improve the cervical mucus have failed,
   HMG may be useful.

Administration

HMG is usually begun between cycle days 2 and 5 at an initial
dose of 1-3 ampules per day. A progestin-induced withdrawal bleed
or a normal menses may be used to time the initiation of HMG. The
dose and duration of therapy depend upon the E_2 response and the
number of follicles recruited. Cervical mucus evaluation provides a
bioassay for the rising levels of E_2. Close monitoring of
individual response is required in HMG administration. Usually 2
ampules per day are given starting on cycle day 3 and a serum E_2
and ultrasound are obtained after 3 days of administration. HMG is
continued at a dose of 2 ampules or greater per day depending on the
patient's response. An E_2 window of 600-1500 pg/ml is sought, with
at least one follicle of 16 mm mean diameter demonstrated on
ultrasound scan on the day of HCG administration. HCG (5000-10,000
I.U.s) is administered by intramuscular injection 24-36 hours after
the last dose of HMG and intercourse is advised 24-36 hours after
the HCG injection. HCG (1500-3000 I.U.) may be administered during
the luteal phase for further support of the corpus luteum if needed.

Complications

Ovarian hyperstimulation syndrome is a potentially fatal
complication of HMG therapy. This condition is a consequence of
multiple follicular development and luteinization. Although the
risk of hyperstimulation syndrome increases with increasing E_2
levels, this condition has also been seen with low E_2 concentrations.
Ovarian hyperstimulation syndrome is rare if the ovulatory dose of
HCG is withheld.

Severe hyperstimulation syndrome may occur in conceptual or
nonceptual cycles and can induce ascites, pleural effusion,
electrolyte imbalance, hypovolemia, hemoconcentration, oliguria,
shock, and thromboembolism. In the severe form, hyperstimulation
syndrome occurs 3-10 days after HCG injection, and ovarian diameters
of greater than 12 cm are found.

156

Cost

HMG is very expensive and now costs between $25.00 and $30.00 per ampule. Patients, therefore, may spend several hundred dollars each month just on the drug.

Outcome

Ovulation can be induced in over 90% of women treated with HMG and pregnancy rates approach 50%. The risk of multiple births is approximately 25% with the majority of these being twin gestations. The risk of spontaneous abortion is 20-25% and some authors have noted an increased risk of ectopic pregnancy.

4. HUMAN URINARY FOLLICLE STIMULATING HORMONE (FSH)

FSH is now commercially available and used both for ovulation induction and for follicular stimulation in patients admitted for in vitro fertilization/embryo transfer. Each vial contains 75 I.U.s of FSH and less than 1 I.U. of LH. Monitoring is essentially the same as with HMG and consists of serum E_2 levels as well as ultrasonography. HCG 5000-10,000 I.U.s are given when the mean follicular diameter of the largest follicle exceeds 16 mm. The complications are also similar to those seen with Pergonal administration and include multiple gestations as well as the chance of hyperstimulation syndrome.

Indications

FSH is indicated for ovulation induction in the patient with chronic anovulation associated with increased LH:FSH ratio typical of that seen in patients with polycystic ovarian syndrome. CC is still the initial drug of choice in these patients, however, FSH may be useful in these patients who do not respond to CC. FSH is also indicated in patients undergoing hyperstimulation protocols for IVF/ET when endogenous LH activity is present.

5. BROMOCRIPTINE (PARLODEL)

Bromocriptine is an ergot alkaloid and dopamine agonist which inhibits pituitary release of prolactin. Bromocriptine is the drug of choice for women with anovulation or luteal phase inadequacy caused by hyperprolactinemia.

Bromocriptine is administered orally starting at a dose of 1.25 mg daily and increasing until the prolactin level is found to be within the normal range. With bromocriptine therapy, restoration of

157

menses occurs in 90% of women within 6-8 weeks and ovulation is
established in over 80% of subjects. A pregnancy rate of 54% is
reported in these patients.

In patients who do not become ovulatory with suppression of the
prolactin level, CC may be indicated.

Bromocriptine is discontinued once the diagnosis of pregnancy
is established. However, should problems develop from enlargement
of a prolactin-secreting pituitary adenoma during pregnancy,
bromocriptine may be reinstituted for control of tumor growth.

6. GONADOTROPIN RELEASING HORMONE (GnRH)

Structure: GnRH is a decapeptide which is synthesized and
secreted by hypothalamic neurons whose nuclei are principally
located in the arcuate nucleus.

Physiology: GnRH is released into the hypothalamic-pituitary-
portal circulation in an episodic manner, with pulses occurring
every 90-120 minutes.

Indications

    Hypothalamic Amenorrhea
        Stress
        Weight loss (weight gain should be encouraged first)
        Anorexia
        Exercise
        Chronic anovulation
        Polycystic ovarian syndrome (in patients unresponsive to CC)
        Hyperprolactinemic anovulation (if Parlodel is poorly
          tolerated or unsuccessful)
        Idiopathic

Administration

    Pulsatile GnRH induces ovulation by stimulating pulsatile
pituitary gonadotropin release. Feedback mechanisms are intact and
ovulation can be induced without the administration of exogenous HCG
and without expensive and complex monitoring.

    GnRH can be administered subcutaneously or intravenously. The
dose required to induce ovulation is higher when given
subcutaneously when compared to the intravenous route, however, it
is easier to maintain access to the subcutaneous tissue than it is
to maintain access intravenously. Most authors report doses of

15-20 µg per pulse given every 90 minutes to induce ovulation when administered subcutaneously, and doses of 25-100 ng/kg per bolus (approximately 3-5 µg per pulse) every 90 minutes when the drug is administered intravenously. Follicular development during GnRH stimulations can be monitored by ultrasonography, cervical mucus examinations, and serum E_2.

Protocol for administering GnRH intravenously (based on using a model AS6H infusion pump [Auto Syringe]):

1. Calculate the patients body weight in kilograms (divide weight in pounds by 2.2).

2. Calculate the dosage of drug to be administered at each bolus (usually every 90 minutes) based on the patients body weight.

3. Mix the drug with diluent to attain the desired concentration (usually 100 µg/ml).

4. Adjust the settings on the Auto Syringe pump to the desired time interval for bolus injections and to the desired dosage for each bolus.

5. Find an appropriate vein in the hand or arm to start the intravenous solution (IV). A small, specially designed 27 gauge needle or intracath may be used. The area for the IV solution must be cleaned carefully with Betadine to ensure a sterile field. Once the IV line is in place, a clear plastic occlusive bandage should be placed over the IV line to help maintain sterility.

6. Once the IV line is in place, attach the tubing to the syringe containing the GnRH and clear the line. Make sure a fresh battery is in the pump and that the pump is working properly.

7. The patient should be cautioned about being careful with the IV line, however, she can go about most of her daily activities without any problem (with the excetion of washing dishes - most patients are glad to give this up). They should keep the IV site clean and dry, but may still bathe without difficulty.

Monitoring

1. The patient should be seen every 2-3 days during the period of stimulation.

2. At each visit do the following:

    a. Cervical mucus check.
    b. Serum E_2: This does not need to be assayed at each visit and may be examined in retrospect.
    c. Review the basal body temperature chart.
    d. Obtain an ultrasound at each visit to determine the number and size of the developing follicles.
    e. Check the syringe to determine if any GnRH needs to be added.
    f. Change the battery at each visit (we use a set of rechargable batteries).
    g. Check the IV site for signs of infection or infiltration. If suspicious, change the IV. With good care, most patients can go 5-7 days with the same IV.

3. When ovulation appears to be imminent, monitor urinary LH.

4. Once ovulation has occurred, support the luteal phase by one of the following methods:

    a. Continue pulsatile GnRH administration throughout the luteal phase (most patients are ready to get rid of the pump at this point).
    b. HCG 2500 I.U.s every 3 days for 3 doses after ovulation.
    c. Progesterone vaginal suppositories 25 mg twice a day.

RESULTS

Patients with hypothylamic amenorrhea have been reported to ovulate between 80 and 100% of the time. Pregnancy rates of 50-80% have been reported in appropriately selected subjects.

Complications

    Subcutaneous administration
      Poor absorption
      Decreased effectiveness
    Intravenous administration
      Discomfort at the injection site
      Thrombophlebitis
    Multiple gestation
    Hyperstimulation
    Development of antibodies to GnRH

SUGGESTED READING

Adashi EY: Clomiphene citrate: mechanism(s) and site(s) of action - a hypothesis revisited. Fertil Steril 42:331, 1984

Daly DC, Walters CA, Soto-Albors CE, Tohan N, Riddick DH: A randomized study of dexamethasone in ovulation induction with clomiphene citrate. Fertil Steril 41:844, 1984

Hammond MG: Monitoring techniques for improved pregnancy rates during clomiphene ovulation induction. Fertil Steril 42:499, 1984

Hammond MG, Halme JK, Talbert LM: Factors affecting the pregnancy rate in clomiphene citrate induction of ovulation. Obstet Gynecol 62:196, 1983

Haning RV Jr, Strawn EY, Nolten WE: Pathophysiology of the ovarian hyperstimulation syndrome. Obstet Gynecol 66:220, 1985

Leyendecker G, Wildt L: Induction of ovulation with chronic intermittent (pulsatile) administration of GnRH in women with hypothalamic amenorrhea. J Reproduc Fertil 69:397, 1983

Oelsner G, Serr DM, Mashiach S, Blankstein J, Snyder M, Lunenfeld B: The study of induction of ovulation with menotropins: analysis of results of 1897 treatment cycles. Fertil Steril 30:538, 1978

Pepperell RJ: A rational approach to ovulation induction. Fertil Steril 40:1, 1983

Schenken RS, Williams RF, Hodgen GD: Ovulation induction using "pure" follicle-stimulating hormone in monkeys. Fertil Steril 41:629, 1984

Schwartz M. Jewelewicz R: The use of gonadotropins for induction of ovulation. Fertil Steril 35:3, 1981

Zacur HA: Ovulation induction with gonadotropin-releasing hormone. Fertil Steril 44:435, 1985

Chapter 13

Male Factor Infertility, Evaluation and Treatment

Carl M. Herbert III, M.D.
B. Jane Rogers, Ph.D.

Infertility is related to a male factor in approximately 40% of infertile couples and to a combined male/female factor in approximately 10%. However, in couples with secondary infertility, only 20% of infertility is due to a male factor alone. Maximal male fertility occurs around age 24-25 years after which there is a slight decrease and then a relatively constant fertilization potential thereafter.

The male partner of an infertile couple warrants evaluation after the couple has attempted to conceive for at least 1 year. Suggestions that a male factor may be involved include an abnormal semen analysis, an abnormal postcoital test (PCT) despite normal cervical mucus, and/or unexplained infertility. The establishment of a diagnosis is extremely important in all forms of infertility including male infertility. The establishment of a diagnosis allows not only an explanation for the infertile condition, but a proper choice of alternatives for therapy and an ability to give a reasonable prognosis for future fertility.

Basic Anatomy and Physiology

A normal ejaculate capable of fertilizing a female is dependent on the normal function of testes and accessory male organs. These are dependent on normal function of an intact hypothalamic-pituitary-gonadal axis. Follicular stimulating hormone (FSH) and luteinizing hormone (LH) play an important role in the initiation of spermatogenesis and in the normal division and maturation of spermatogonia becoming healthy spermatozoa.

LH stimulates the Leydig cells to produce testosterone which has a high local concentration in the gonad and acts on the accessory male organs to ensure the production of adequate secretions and the normal maturation of sperm during their movement through the epididymis. At ejaculation, mature spermatozoa from the vas deferens are joined by secretions from the seminal vesicles and the prostate gland. The initial emission usually contains the majority of the spermatozoa in the ejaculate and the subsequent secretions are more from accessory sex organs. FSH binds to the Sertoli cells to stimulate spermatogenesis and production of androgen-binding protein and inhibin. Inhibin exerts a negative feedback effect on FSH output by the pituitary.

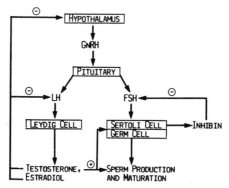

A summary of the important components in the male reproductive system is shown below:

Seminiferous Tubules

85% of testis
Total length 0.9 miles
Sertoli cells for production
    of nutrients, androgen
    binding protein, inhibin
Spermatogonia
Maintenance of blood-testis
    barrier

Spermatogenesis

70-90 days for sperm
    development
Induced by FSH
Maintained by testosterone

Epididymis

20-30 days for sperm transport
Acquire motility and capacity
    for fertilization

Seminal Vesicles

Fructose secreted

Prostate

Liquefaction

Sperm maturation is a process taking between 70 and 90 days, therefore, after a testicular insult or initiating therapy, change in the semen analysis is not expected before 2-3 months.

Etiologies of Male Infertility

Selection of appropriate therapy depends upon the accurate establishment of a diagnosis. One classification system for the etiologies of male infertility is based on semen abnormalities (Reproduced by permission by G.S. Bernstein, Male Factor in Reproduction, Endocrinology, Infertility, and Contraception, Medical Econcomics Books, Oradell, NJ 1986, 436).

SEMEN PARAMETER	ETIOLOGY
ABNORMAL COUNT AZOOSPERMIA	KLINEFELTER'S SYNDROME OR OTHER GENETIC DISORDERS SERTOLI-CELL-ONLY SYNDROME SEMINIFEROUS TUBULE OR LEYDIG CELL FAILURE HYPOGONADOTROPIC HYPOGONADISM DUCTAL OBSTRUCTION, INCLUDING YOUNG'S SYNDROME VARICOCELE EXOGENOUS FACTORS
OLIGOZOOSPERMIA	GENETIC DISORDER ENDOCRINOPATHIES, INCUDING ANDROGEN RECEPTOR DEFECTS VARICOCELE AND OTHER ANATOMIC DISORDERS MATURATION ARREST HYPOSPERMATOGENESIS EXOGENOUS FACTORS
ABNORMAL VOLUME NO EJACULATE	DUCTAL OBSTRUCTION RETROGRADE EJACULATION EJACULATORY FAILURE HYPOGANDISM
LOW VOLUME	OBSTRUCTION OF EJACULATORY DUCTS ABSENCE OF SEMINAL VESICLES AND VAS DEFERENS PARTIAL RETROGRADE EJACULATION INFECTION
HIGH VOLUME	UNKNOWN FACTORS
ABNORMAL MOTILITY	IMMUNOLOGIC FACTORS INFECTION VARICOCELE DEFECTS IN SPERM STRUCTURE METABOLIC OR ANATOMIC ABNORMALTIES OF SPERM POOR LIQUEFACTION OF SEMEN
ABNORMAL VISCOSITY	ETIOLOGY UNKNOWN
ABNORMAL MORPHOLOGY	VARICOCELE STRESS INFECTION EXOGENOUS FACTORS UNKNOWN FACTORS
EXTRANEOUS CELLS	INFECTION OR INFLAMMATION SHEDDING OF IMMATURE SPERM

The following classification of the causes of male oligospermia takes into consideration the sperm count and a measurement of serum FSH (Paulson, 1978). Testosterone and LH values are sometimes measured although they are only occasionally helpful.

ETIOLOGY OF OLIGOSPERMIA

	FSH	LH	T	ABNORMALITIES
PREGERMINAL	↓ OR NL	NL	NL	HYPOPITUITARISM HYPOTHYROIDISM GLUCOCORTICOID EXCESS ANDROGEN EXCESS ESTROGEN EXCESS SYSTEMIC DISEASES (DIABETES) VARICOCELE DRUGS
GERMINAL	↑	NL OR ↑	NL OR ↓	CHROMOSOMAL ABNORMALITIES CRYPTORCHIDISM MATURATION ARREST HYPOSPERMATOGENESIS SERTOLI-CELL-ONLY SYNDROME RADIATION OR CHEMOTHERAPY MUMPS VARICOCELE
POSTGERMINAL	NL	NL	NL	ANATOMIC ABNORMALITIES DUCTAL OBSTRUCTION GENITAL INFECTION IMMUNOLOGIC REACTIONS ABNORMAL SECONDARY SEX GLANDS ERECTILE OR EJACULATORY DISTURBANCES

EVALUATION OF THE MALE

I. History
II. Physical examination
III. Laboratory evaluation
    A. Semen studies
        1. semen analysis
        2. sperm penetration assay (SPA)
        3. antisperm antibody assays (AsAb)
        4. mucus penetration tests
        5. hyperosmotic swelling test (HOS)
        6. computerized motility evaluation
    B. Blood studies
        1. LH, FSH, testosterone, prolactin
        2. hypothalamic-pituitary tests
        3. karyotype
    C. Radiology studies
        1. ultrasound (Doppler)
        2. vasography
        3. pituitary CT scan

I. History

A careful history should be taken including consideration of the following:

1. Present or past illnesses or disease states (mumps orchitis, severe metabolic or nutritional diseases, chronic or hereditary illnesses).
2. Trauma, surgery, radiation, chemotherapy, or infectious damage to the genitals.
3. Current medications, smoking, alcohol ingestion, recreational drug use.
4. Occupational or environmental exposures.
5. Sexual history including coital techniques, erectile and ejaculatory function.
6. History of fertility with other partners.
7. Family history of infertility or genital surgery.

II. Physical Examination

A general physical examination should be accomplished looking for any obvious abnormalities. Special attention should be directed to body hair distribution, evidence of gynecomastia, weight, and blood pressure. Examination of the genitalia should include an evaluation of penile length, location and formation of the urethral meatus, pubic hair development, size and consistency of the testis, presence or absence of a varicocele, the size and consistency of the prostate gland.

Cryptorchidism is lack of proper descent of one or both testicles. This is seen in 3-4% of newborn males and less than 1% of males by the age of 1 year. An orchiopexy is recommended before age 2 years because of progressive impairment and infertility. When the testicle is brought into the scrotum prior to puberty, 30-62% are fertile compared to only 13-46% when surgery is delayed until later life. However, the etiology for an undescended testicle may also ultimately influence sperm production and, therefore, correcting the anatomical location may not change the future fertility of some males. The risk of malignancy in an undescended testicle whether replaced into the scrotum or left intra-abdominal is increased and regular evaluation is recommended.

III. Laboratory Evaluation

Semen Studies:

The semen analysis is still the mainstay for diagnosis of male infertility. Considerable variation may occur from one semen analysis to another and, therefore, frequently several semen analyses are necessary before a definitive diagnosis can be accomplished. It is important that a laboratory experienced in evaluation of semen is chosen to avoid inaccurate results and a report of "normal" is inadequate.

After at least 2 days and preferably less than 5 days abstinence, a masturbatory specimen is collected in a clean jar and brought to the laboratory within 60 minutes. The sample is allowed to liquefy at 37°C and then examined for the following parameters:

A. Count. Sperm concentration of 20-250 million sperm/ml is normal. Oligozoospermia represents less than 20 million sperm/ml. Azoospermia defines complete absence of sperm in the ejaculate. The total number of sperm per ejaculate which is considered abnormal is still controversial but ranges from below 20 to 80 million.

B. Volume. Normal is 2-6 ml, although 2-3 ml is average. Increased or decreased seminal volume may produce inadequate fertility. Concentration of sperm by split ejaculate or centrifugation can be used for large volumes and washing and dilution may be appropriate for small volumes with high counts.

C. Motility. Greater than 50% is considered normal. Progressive motility of the majority of the sample is assessed subjectively on a 0-4 scale with 3-4 considered normal. Absence of motility and viability (proven by a live/dead stain) is called necrospermia. A semen analysis with less than 40% motile sperm represents asthenozoospermia.

D. Morphology. Greater than 50% normal forms is considered adequate. Every normal ejaculate has a substantial portion of abnormal forms present. These abnormal forms may include macrocephalic, microcephalic, amorphous, tapered, immature, and tail defective sperm. The absolute association of any one sperm form with a fertility impairment (such as increased tapered forms with a varicocele) is controversial. However, the predominance of abnormal forms is a clear indicator of faulty spermatogenesis and decreased fertility.

E. Liquefaction. A normal ejaculate should liquefy within 20-30 minutes of collection. Poor liquefaction may result from enzyme deficiencies in the seminal plasma in turn reflecting an abnormality of the seminal vesicles. Although still unproven, the addition of amylase or other proteolytic enzymes may be beneficial. Ejaculation into culture medium is an alternative approach.

F. pH. pH should be slightly alkaline (7.2-7.8). Timing of pH measurement can cause variation and should be done as soon after collection as possible.

G. Viscosity. Normal viscosity of completely liquefied semen should be slightly greater than that of serum. Viscosity is rated as 1-4 with 1 as highly viscous and 4 as watery. Normal values would be 2-3. The relevance of either increased or decreased viscosity on fertility is unknown.

H. Sperm Agglutination and/or Aggregation. Slight agglutination can be normal but moderate or heavy agglutination is undesirable. Agglutination defines sperm sticking to other sperm while aggregation defines sperm sticking to other material. Heavy agglutination may reflect the presence of antisperm antibodies while heavy aggregation may indicate genital tract infection.

I. Round Cells (Leukocytes and Sperm Precursors). When greater than 2 million round cells/ml of ejaculate are detected, differential staining is indicated. Utilizing a peroxidase stain, the leukocytes will stain positively while the immature sperm forms will not. Leukocytosis is indicative of infection, most frequently prostatitis, and may require antibiotic therapy. Large numbers of sperm precursors are indicative of defective spermatogenesis and may not be amenable to therapy.

J. Particulate Debris. Large amounts of debris in a semen analysis may inhibit fertility. Detection of this in a semen analysis may be an indication for a "swim-up" or a "rise" technique to allow insemination with motile sperm avoiding the other detrimental material.

Performance of a classic semen analysis involves the following:

1. Collection. The sample is collected by masturbation into a sterile container. If the patient cannot collect a masturbatory specimen, special nonspermicidal silastic condoms can be used during intercourse. The time of collection, time of abstinence, and spillage should be noted when the sample is given to the laboratory.

2. Gross Physical Examination. Record liquefaction time, viscosity, color, volume, ph, and presence of persistent gel after 30 minutes.

3. <u>Microscopic Examination</u>. Place an aliquot of raw semen on a slide, <u>cover with a cover slip</u>, and examine at low power (10X) for motility, presence of agglutination or aggregation, particulate debris, and round cells. Quantitative motility can be done using a hemocytometer or computer assisted analysis.

4. <u>Morphology</u>. Prepare two smears of fresh semen mixed with eosin-nigrosin stain, air dry, do morphology at 100X magnification with an oil emersion lens. Examine 100-200 sperm recording percent of abnormal forms of each type. Do peroxidase stain if round cells are of significant concentration.

5. <u>Sperm Count</u>. Diluted counts can be made using a Newbauer hemocytometer or undiluted counts can be made using a Makler chamber. The extent of dilution is determined based on the "guestimate" made during the original microscopic examination. A 1:10 dilution is appropriate for most samples in the normal range. Very low concentrations (less than 5 million/ml) should be diluted 1 to 5 or 1:2. Count the four corner squares on a hemocytometer and the middle square of a 25 square grid. The concentration/ml can be calculated as follows:

$$\text{count/ml} = \frac{\text{count/sq} \times \text{dilution factor}}{\text{hemocytometer factor}}$$

Sperm Penetration Assay (SPA)

As fertility and infertility have been documented over a broad range of semen parameters, a test for sperm function has been sought to augment the descriptive statistics obtained from a semen analysis. The first such test developed was one to measure the ability of sperm penetration into the egg. The best test of human sperm penetration is into a normal human egg. However, due to moral, ethical, and logistical considerations, a human egg penetration test is not available. Only recently during cycles of in vitro fertilization has it been possible to assess human sperm-human egg penetration and fertilization. However, a method using zona-free hamster eggs has been developed which can assay the penetration ability of human sperm.

Correlation of the results of SPAs with fertility has shown that penetration of 10% or more of the hamster eggs is compatible with a fertile ejaculate. Penetration of less than 10% of the hamster eggs may indicate reduced or absent fertilizing capability. It should be remembered that this is a bioassay and the variations and potential problems of a bioassay frequently require repetitive testing before making a final diagnosis. For example, combined

studies during in vitro fertilization attempts have shown that up to
15% of men capable of penetrating their wife's eggs will obtain an
abnormal result while trying to penetrate hamster eggs.
Nevertheless, the SPA has given us the first measure of the
physiologic function of sperm and is an important adjunct in the
evaluation of male infertility.

THE SPERM PENETRATION ASSAY

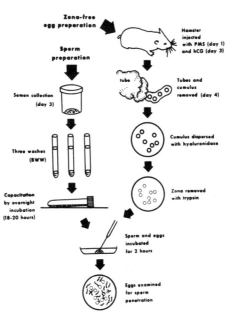

A modification of the SPA, use of a TEST-yolk buffer, has been
developed. This buffered nutrient broth is used for sperm shipped
by mail for testing in laboratories distant from collection sites.
This broth contains: ultrafiltered water, TES buffer, Tris buffer,
chicken egg yolk, fructose or D-Glucose, and antibiotics (Pen/Strep).
Sperm incubated in this TEST-yolk buffer have been found to have
increased motility and increased ability to penetrate in the SPA.
The percent penetration considered normal with TEST-yolk buffer in
our laboratory is twice that without buffer or 20%.

Antisperm Antibody (AsAb) Assays

Indications for AsAb assays include poor sperm-mucus
interaction with "shivering sperm" phenomenon, the presence of sperm
agglutination in a semen analysis, and otherwise unexplained
infertility. The most common etiology for male AsAb is reversal of
a previous vasectomy. AsAb may be detected in the serum of the male
and/or female, in the mucus of the female, or in the semen of the
male. AsAb have been classified as agglutinating, immobilizing, and
cytotoxic. However, the significance of antisperm antibodies in the
prevention of fertilization and pregnancy has not yet been well
defined. The following is a list of tests used to detect antisperm
antibodies:

TESTS TO DETECT ANTISPERM ANTIBODIES

SPERM AGGLUTINATION			
GELATIN AGGLUTINATION	KIBRICK	}	IG G
MICROAGGLUTINATION	FRANKLIN–DUKES		IG M
TRAY AGGLUTINATION	FRIBERG		IG A
COMPLEMENT DEPENDENT			
IMMOBILIZATION	ISOJIMA	}	IG G
CYTOTOXIC	CYTOTOX		IG M
MIXED AGGLUTINATION REACTION	MAR		IG G
IMMUNOBEAD BINDING	IMMUNOBEAD		IG G
			IG M
			IG A

A significant improvement in the area of antisperm antibodies
is the immunobead reaction. This allows detection of specific
subclasses of antibodies (IgA, IgG, IgM) and specific locations for
sperm binding (head, midpiece, tail). Hopefully, this methodology
will improve the evaluation of AsAb and their effects on fertility.

(Reproduced by permission
Clarke GN et al Am J
Reproduc Immunol 7:20, 1985).

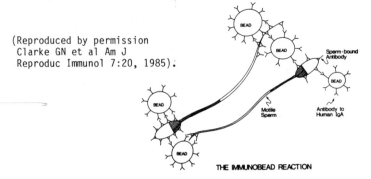

THE IMMUNOBEAD REACTION

Mucus Penetration Tests

Mucus penetration tests can be divided into two major classes,
(1) in vivo - PCT or (2) in vitro - mucus penetration on a slide or
in a tube. Abnormalities in mucus penetration may be related to
either abnormal sperm or abnormal mucus. To evaluate the
contribution of both, mucus penetration testing is performed by
cross-matching sperm and mucus from the couple being investigated
and donor sperm and donor mucus. Donor mucus may be human,
synthetic, or bovine mucus. A four-way cross-match testing should
be performed as described below.

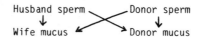

Interpretation of this testing is somewhat subjective and must be
standardized in an individual laboratory.

Hyperosmotic Swelling HOS Tests

Rationale for the HOS test derives from knowledge that
spermatozoa with functional (biochemically active) membranes will
increase in volume when exposed to a hyposmotic medium. This medium
exerts an osmotic stress that is great enough to cause an influx of
water without causing lysis of the membrane. The increasing volume
is detected in the tail area of the sperm as expansion of sperm
membranes causes curling of the tail fibers. The assay monitors
curling sperm tails, and if a sperm swells in the HOS test, it is
considered normal. Interpretation of this test requires the
evaluation of 100 sperm with more than 60% curling tailed sperm
being considered normal and less than 50% abnormal. The data to
date show the percentage of spermatozoa which swell correlates well
with the in vitro penetrating capability of the spermatozoa in an
SPA. This test, therefore, may be a reliable indicator of the
outcome of human in vitro fertilization and avoid the variability of
a semen analysis.

Computerized Motility Evaluation

The advent of microcomputers has made it possible to measure
objectively the detailed movement characteristics of human
spermatozoa. These techniques allow determination of the percentage
of motile sperm, their average speed, the frequency distribution of
their velocities, and other quantitative motility parameters such as
linearity and lateral head displacement. Parameters for normality
are still being defined with this technology but at present sperm
velocity for the majority of sperm in a specimen should be greater

than 25 ug/second. The advantage of this technology is its unbiased reproducibility without observer variation. The negative aspects of these studies are the expense of the equipment ($15,000 to $45,000) and lack of standardization for infertility parameters.

Blood Studies

Gross abnormalities in spermatogenesis and testicular function may be detected by measuring serum gonadotropins and testosterone levels. The negative feedback system between the testes and hypothalamic-pituitary axis allows a differential diagnosis to be made between primary testicular damage and abnormalities of the neuroregulating factors. An elevated prolactin should be suspected when an element of impotence is associated with male infertility. Hypothalamic pituitary testing utilizing GnRH and other releasing factors has only limited applicability in the management of most infertile males. A peripheral karyotype can be helpful especially in males with extremely low sperm counts and elevated gonadotropins. A chromosomal abnormality has been found in 2% of men with a sperm concentration $< 20 \times 10^6$/ml. However, the frequency of an abnormal karyotype is increased with a decreased sperm concentration and 20% of men who are with a sperm concentration of $< 1 \times 10^6$/ml were found to have a genetic abnormality. The most common genetic abnormality found is Klinefelter's syndrome, 47,XXY.

Radiologic Studies

Ultrasound examination of the male reproductive and urologic system may help define certain abnormalities. Doppler studies have been employed to evaluate small varicoceles. Vasography may be needed for patients with evidence of an obstructed vas, and may allow determination of those men capable of surgical repair. Radiologic pituitary evaluation (CAT scan) is important especially in men with elevated prolactin. Pituitary tumors can decrease gonadotropin output, increase prolactin output, and therefore, be associated with infertility.

Treatment of Male Infertility

Treatment modalities for male infertility remain controversial. Nevertheless, a systematic approach to the diagnosis of male factor infertility may optimize the possibility for successful therapy. Utilizing the following algorithms, some direction for treatment of various diagnoses can be achieved.

Complete absence of sperm in the ejaculate, azoospermia, is frequently untreatable. An elevated FSH signifies germinal failure and no further treatment or work-up is indicated. A low FSH may

reflect hypothalamic pituitary dysfunction and evaluation continues
as it would for an oligospermic infertility patient. In the
presence of a normal FSH, ductile obstruction and retrograde
ejaculation must be ruled out. The detection of fructose in the
semen indicates the presence of seminal vesicles and a patent distal
vas deferens.

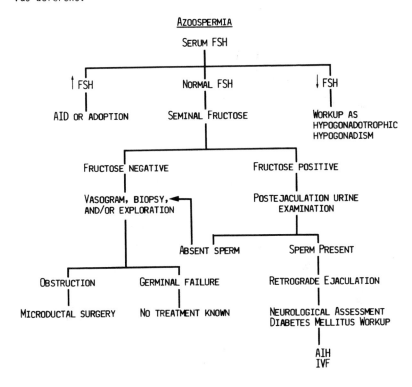

An ejaculate with less than 40% motile sperm, asthenospermia,
but normal sperm numbers may reflect infection, medication, toxins,
AsAb, or an idiopathic condition. More frequently, low motility is
found in association with low sperm concentration and is evaluated
under oligospermia.

174

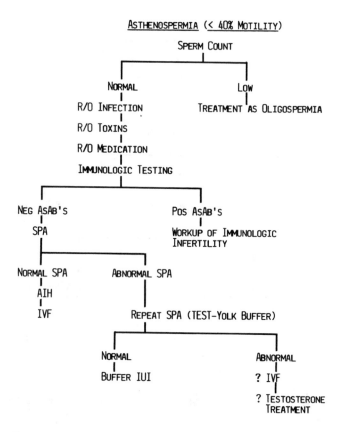

ASTHENOSPERMIA (< 40% MOTILITY)

SPERM COUNT

NORMAL
R/O INFECTION
R/O TOXINS
R/O MEDICATION
IMMUNOLOGIC TESTING

LOW
TREATMENT AS OLIGOSPERMIA

NEG ASAB'S
SPA

POS ASAB'S
WORKUP OF IMMUNOLOGIC INFERTILITY

NORMAL SPA
AIH
IVF

ABNORMAL SPA

REPEAT SPA (TEST-YOLK BUFFER)

NORMAL
BUFFER IUI

ABNORMAL
? IVF
? TESTOSTERONE TREATMENT

The most common abnormality on a semen analysis of an infertile male is reduction in the sperm count, oligospermia. Oligospermia is usually defined as less than 20 million sperm/ml and less 60 million total sperm per ejaculate. In most men with oligospermia, motility and morphology are also affected. It should be remembered, however, that a single semen analysis is not adequate to make a diagnosis of oligospermia secondary to the considerable intrapatient variability and the frequency of collection problems.

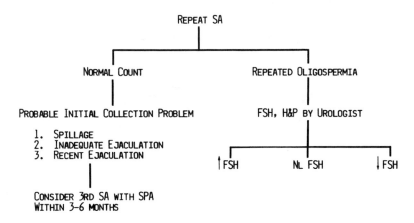

OLIGOSPERMIA ($\leq$20 x 10^{6}SPERM/ML)

REPEAT SA

NORMAL COUNT   REPEATED OLIGOSPERMIA

PROBABLE INITIAL COLLECTION PROBLEM   FSH, H&P BY UROLOGIST

1. SPILLAGE
2. INADEQUATE EJACULATION
3. RECENT EJACULATION

↑FSH   NL FSH   ↓FSH

CONSIDER 3RD SA WITH SPA
WITHIN 3-6 MONTHS

Oligospermia with low gonadotropins reflects hypogonadotropic hypogonadism. An elevated prolactin level in this setting supports a pituitary tumor. Inadequate gonadotropin production is most commonly Kallmann's syndrome (with impaired olfaction) but isolated LH and FSH deficiences have been reported. Some unusual syndromes including Prader-Willi and Laurence-Moon-Biedl present with abnormal pubescence.

Oligospermia with elevated gonadotropins implies some degree of primary testicular damage. Clinically, these patients seem to fall into two categories, those with are severe oligospermia and marked elevation of FSH and those with mild oligospermia and only mild elevations of FSH. Those patients with severe oligospermia or azoospermia may have a genetic etiology such as Klinefelter's syndrome or a form of gonadal dysgenesis. Therefore, they should have a peripheral karyotype done. Regardless, an elevated FSH eliminates the use of medications whose method of action is elevation of gonadotropins (i.e., Clomid, Tamoxifen).

Oligospermic males with normal FSH values constitute the largest portion of infertile males. Traditionally these men have first been evaluated for the presence of a varicocele and then treated with medical therapy if one was not found. With the advent of the SPA and the equivocal results after varicocelectomies, we have chosen to use the SPA as an initial evaluating mechanism before considering therapy.

REPEATED OLIGOSPERMIA, NORMAL FSH

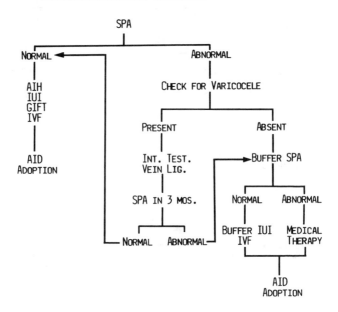

Modalities of Therapy

Unfortunately, clinical studies evaluating the efficacy of different modalities of therapy for male infertility have frequently been inadequate. These studies are often not performed in a blinded or controlled fashion; do not have uniform definitions and/or diagnostic criteria; use a variety of different medicine doses and regimens for varying lengths of time; and fail to use the delivery of a viable infant as a true measure of success. Other problems include failure to evaluate the female partner adequately; failure to evaluate the male fully before placing him within a diagnostic category; and drawing conclusions from very small patient samples. As a result, statistics on the percentage of "improvement" and pregnancies for a particular therapy have frequently been reported over a broad range making it difficult to predict potential outcome for the individual patient. An example of this confusion is found in the management of the varicocele.

Varicocele is an abnormal dilatation of the pampiniform plexus of the internal spermatic vein. Its incidence among infertile males is 20-40% in most reported series. This is two to three times higher than the incidence of varicoceles in the general male population. Theories regarding the mechanism of infertility secondary to a varicocele center around venostasis or reflux in the dilated testicular vein. This change in blood flow is thought potentially to elevate the testicular temperature; or cause reflux of adrenal and renal metabolytes which are toxic to the testicle; or to cause a relative hypoxia secondary to venostasis. Although the reflux and stasis have been documented on venography, there are no data to confirm the speculations on exact pathophysiology. Similarly, the "stress-pattern" which was described as an increase in the number of tapered sperm with an overall decrease in motility and a variable change in sperm concentration has been found to be present in men with alcohol abuse or following a high fever as well as in those displaying a varicocele. A wide range of sperm parameters has been documented in males with varicoceles making a particular abnormal parameter less meaningful. Nevertheless, after therapy with surgical ligation or radiologic occlusion of the internal spermatic vein, studies have reported improved semen quality in 50-90% of treated men. Conception rates, however, have been far lower than this ranging 25-50%. Very recent studies using life table analysis and control subjects have failed to show an increase in pregnancy rate for most men undergoing a varicocelectomy. This therapeutic modality for male infertility like many others requires more investigation to determine which men if any would most likely benefit from this procedure for treatment of their infertility.

Preejaculatory Systemic Medical Therapy

Any chronic or acute medical illness should be identified and properly treated (i.e., CAH). However, the common practice of administering thyroid hormone to infertile men is of no benefit in the absence of thyroid disease. Success with medical therapies is most likely to occur if a single treatable cause for infertility can be identified. The most common forms of medical therapy are shown on the next page.

PREEJACULATION SYSTEMIC MEDICAL THERAPIES

MEDICINE	DOSE	INDICATION	MECHANISM OF ACTION	PROBLEMS
CLOMIPHENE CITRATE	25-50 MG PO QD	OLIGOSPERMIA	INCREASE FSH	PARADOXICAL SPERM SUPPRESSION
TAMOXIFEN	10-20 MG PO QD	OLIGOSPERMIA	INCREASE FSH	PARADOXICAL SPERM SUPPRESSION
TESTOSTERONE ENANTHATE	20 MG IM Q WEEK	SEVERE OLIGOSPERMIA	REBOUND FROM SUPPRESSION OF FSH	PERSISTANCE OF SUPPRESSION, AZOOSPERMIA
FLUOXYMESTERONE	5 MG PO BID	ASTHENOSPERMIA	INCREASE INTRATESTICULAR TESTOSTERONE	ELEVATED HEPATIC ENZYMES, SPERM SUPPRESSION
GNRH	25 MCG/KG SQ Q 120 MIN. VIA PUMP	HYPOGONADOTROPIC HYPOGONADISM	INCREASE PIT. LH/FSH OUTPUT	CONSTANT INFUSION
HMG PLUS HCG	½-1 AMPULE IM 3x/WEEK, 2000 IU IM 3x/WEEK	HYPOGONADOTROPHIC HYPOGONADISM	INITIATE SPERMATOGENESIS WITH LH/FSH	MAY TAKE 6-12 MONTHS, EXPENSIVE
HCG ALONE	2000-5000 IU IM 2-3x/WEEK	OLIGOASTHENOSPERMIA ADJUNCT TO VARICOCELECTOMY	INCREASE SERUM AND INTRATESTICULAR TESTOSTERONE	PARADOXICAL SPERM SUPPRESSION
GLUCOCORTICOIDS METHYLPREDNISOLONE	32 MG PO TID INTERMITTENT TAPERING DOSES EACH CYCLE	ANTISPERM ANTIBODIES	IMMUNE SUPPRESSION	MOOD CHANGES, PEPTIC ULCERS, ASEPTIC NECROSIS (HEAD OF FEMUR)
PREDNISONE	5 MG PO BID/TID, 10-20 MG PO QOD, CONTINUOUSLY	ANTISPERM ANTIBODIES	IMMUNE SUPPRESSION	SAME
ANTIBIOTICS TRIMETHOPRIM/ SULFAMETHOXAZOLE	1 DS TABLET PO BID	PYOSPERMIA/PROSTATITIS	ANTIBIOTIC	RARE
DOXYCYCLINE	100 MG PO QD/BID	PYOSPERMIA/PROSTATITIS	ANTIBIOTIC	PHOTOSENSITIVITY, NAUSEA

Postejaculatory Mechanical Sperm Treatment

Postejaculatory mechanical treatment involves a combination of the following insemination techniques and sperm treatments.

Insemination Techniques	Sperm Treatments
Intravaginal	Split Ejaculate
Cervical (Mylex Cup)	Sperm Wash
Intracervical	Sperm Rise
Intrauterine	Incubation in Therapeutic Media

Intravaginal insemination is easily accomplished at home and requires little technical assistance. Cervical insemination techniques using a Mylex cup require proper size selection and allow sperm to avoid a potentially hostile vaginal milieu. Intracervical and intrauterine inseminations require the technical assistance of a laboratory to separate sperm from the semen and to avoid the problems of uterine cramping and rarely anaphylaxis. Sperm treatments may be as simple as obtaining the first portion of a split ejaculate. Seventy-five percent of the spermatozoa are found in the first 40% of the ejaculate in 88% of men. Using this concentrated portion of the ejaculate prevents a potential detrimental dilutional effect. Sperm washing is accomplished by centrifugation in culture media such as Ham's F-10 or BWW media. This technique separates the semen from the sperm. However, a "swim-up" or a "rise" technique will allow separation of the motile from nonmotile sperm. This may allow the sperm with greater fertilization potential to avoid prolonged contact with dead sperm and potentially toxic substances. A number of substances have been thought to be therapeutic or enhancing to sperm. Media containing caffeine, kallikrein, arginine, and most recently TEST-yolk buffer have been utilized in an attempt to improve sperm fertilization capability.

These techniques provide proven benefit for the following conditions:

1. Anatomic defects (hypospadias, chordee, Peyronie's disease)
2. Sexual dysfunction (premature ejaculation, impotence)
3. Retrograde ejaculation (diabetes, spinal injury)

They provide possible benefit in the following conditions:

1. Hypospermia - ejaculate less than 2 ml
2. Hyperspermia - ejaculate greater than 6 ml
3. Polyzoospermia - count greater than 500 million/ml
4. Oligoasthenozoospermia - counts less than 20 million/ml and/or motility less than 40%.

New Technologies

In vitro fertilization (IVF) is playing a small but growing role in the treatment of male infertility. Data to date show a decreased pregnancy rate among male factor in comparison to other etiologies of infertility treated by IVF. The decreased pregnancy rate reflects a decrease in total number of eggs fertilized and, therefore, total number of embryos transferred. Pregnancy rates are equivalent to patients with tubal factor infertility when equal numbers of embryos are transferred. Of the individual semen parameters, only an extreme decrease in motility (less than 20%) is consistently predictive of decreased fertilization. A combination of low motility (<40%), low count (<20 x 10^6/ml), and increased abnormal forms (>50%) also carries a poor prognosis for IVF. Interestingly, men with exceptionally low sperm counts (less than 5 million/ml) whose motility is reasonably normal have a fair chance of fertilizing human eggs in vitro.

Techniques of IVF have created the potential for a more direct form of fertilization, injection of a single spermatozoa into an egg by micromanipulation. This technology is presently available, however, it bypasses the biologic safeguards that may prevent genetically or otherwise abnormal gametes from fusing. Until the proper egg and proper sperm can be identified and other ethical and scientific considerations clarified, this will remain an experimental technique.

Alternatives

Two final options which circumvent a noncorrectable form of male infertility include artificial insemination by donor (AID) and adoption. Over the last several years there have been fewer infants to adopt and more couples desiring to adopt them creating an environment of anxiety and frustration for many couples. One of the results is increased utilization of AID programs. Selection of a well established AID program with rigorous screening criteria is critical secondary to increasing problems with sexually transmitted diseases and increasing numbers of diseases found to have a hereditary component (i.e., hypertension, heart disease, and certain malignancies).

SUGGESTED READING

Allen N, Herbert CM, Maxson WS, Rogers BJ, Diamond MP, Wentz AC: Intrauterine insemination. A critical reviw. Fertil Steril 44:569-580, 1985.

Bernstein GS: Male factor. In Reproductive Endocrinology, Infertility, and Contraception, Oradell, NJ Medical Economics Books, 1986, p. 436.

Bronson R, Cooper G, Rosenfield D: Sperm antibodies: Their role in infertility. Fertil Steril 42:2, 1984.

Cohen J, Edwards R, Fehilly C, Fishel S, Hewitt J, Purdy J, Rowland G, Steptoe P, Webster J: In vitro fertilization: A treatment for female infertility. Fertil Steril 43:422-432, 1985.

Crockett ATK, Netto ICV, Dougherty KA, Urry RL: Semen analysis: A review of samples from 225 men seen in an infertility clinic. J Urol 114:560-563, 1975.

deVere White R, Paulston DF: Staging profile of hypofertile male subjects. J Urol 120:71, 1978.

Kjessler B: Chromosomal constitution and male reporductive failure. In Mancinni RE, Martini L (eds): Male Fertility and Sterility. New York, Academic Press, 1974, pp. 231-274.

LaNasa JA Jr, Urry RL: Evaluation and treatment of the infertile male. Sem Reproduc Endorcrinol 3:113, 1985.

Rogers BJ: The sperm penetration assay: Its usefulness reevaluated. Fertil Steril 43:821, 1985.

Saypol DC: Varicocele. Semin Urol 2:82-90, 1984.

Schellen AMCM: Clomiphene citrate in the treatment of male infertility. In Jain J, Schill WB, Scshwarzstein L (eds.): Treatment of Male Infertility, Berlin, Springer-Verlag, 1982, pp. 33-34.

Van Der Ven HH, Jeyendran RS, Al-Hansani S, Perez-Pelaez M, Diedrich K, Zaneveld LJD: Correlation between human sperm swelling in hypoosmotic medium (hypoosmotic swelling test) and in vitro fertilization. J Androl 7:190-196, 1986.

Vermeulen A, Vandeweghe M, Deslypere JP: Prognosis of subfertility in men with corrected or uncorrected varicocele. J Androl 7:147-155, 1986.

Chapter 14

The Cervical Factor, Evaluation and Therapy

Anne Colston Wentz, M.D.

It is generally accepted that cervical mucus can be a barrier to ascending sperm and that the investigation of sperm-cervical mucus interaction is an integral part of the basic infertility evaluation. Changes in the physical properties of the mucus can also provide information about the hormonal milieu of the patient. Observation of sperm motility in cervical mucus can suggest the presence of antisperm antibodies. Abnormalities of the mucus and of the sperm can both be detected, and a step wise approach is needed to differentiate the various diagnostic possibilities and to treat them appropriately.

DEFINITION. Cervical factor infertility usually implies abnormal sperm-mucus interaction initially discovered by observing a poor postcoital test (PCT). However, a poor PCT may be due to sperm abnormalities and not to the mucus, so the diagnosis is made by exclusion of sperm abnormalities.

INCIDENCE. Cervical factor infertility is estimated in 5-10% of couples. If all forms of abnormal mucus-sperm interactions are included, the incidence is at least 20-30%.

1. Cervical Score: A cervical scoring method allows comparison of estimations of cervical mucus quality and quantity even though performed by different observers. This semiquantitative scoring system is shown.

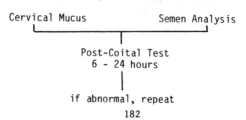

Evaluation of Sperm-Mucus Interaction

Cervical Mucus   Semen Analysis

Post-Coital Test
6 - 24 hours

if abnormal, repeat

CERVICAL SCORE

Parameter Score	0	1	2	3
Amount of mucus	None	Scant	Dribble	Cascade
Spinnbarkeit (cm)	0-2	3-6	7-10	Over 10
Ferning	None	Linear	Partially Branched	Completely Branched
Viscosity	Thick	Medium	Sl.Thin	Very Thin
Cervical Os	Closed	Sl.Dilated	Open	Gaping
Total Score	0	5	10	15

2. Postcoital Examination, Huhner Test (PCT): The PCT and other "performance tests" that will be described are done to identify cervical mucus problems, semen abnormalities, specific sperm-mucus incompatibility, and problems with coital technique.

The cervical mucus is most conducive to sperm survival, transport, and nutrition during the 3 days before ovulation. The stimulation from rising estradiol (E_2) levels will cause mucus to be abundant in quantity, thin, clear, runny, acellular, have a good Spinnbarkeit (up to 12 cm.), and maintain large numbers of adequately motile sperm. Mucus with inadequate estrogen support, or under the influence of progesterone (P_4), is scant, thick, cloudy, gummy, cellular, and will not support sperm penetration or survival.

Patient Instructions: The PCT is an evaluation of sperm survival and motility in cervical mucus. The test is done just before ovulation, usually between days 10 and 14 of the normal cycle. The patient should be asked to have intercourse within 6-24 hours of her office visit. A very short interval between intercourse and the visit is stressful, and gives misleading information about sperm motility. Observation 8-12 hours after intercourse provides better documentation of long-term sperm survival and rules out immunoglobulin-mediated sperm cytotoxicity.

Technique: The patient is placed in the lithotomy position, a speculum inserted, and the cervix visualized. The cervix should be gently wiped clean with a dry sponge. A tuberculin syringe is then inserted (without needle) into the endocervical canal, and the plunger retracted. A Kelly may be used to grasp the mucus at the cervical os, and the Spinnbarkeit tested as the syringe is removed. The thread may stretch to the introitus. If the specimen is inadequate, a second aspiration may be performed. The plastic top is then placed upon the syringe, and the syringe kept safe until examination is possible. Mucus stored in this fashion is virtually airtight and can be used for in vitro studies even the following day.

Examination: The cervical mucus is first examined under low power, and scanned for debris, cells, Trichomonas and Monilia, and for sperm. Its quality and quantity are noted, and a cervical score calculated. The examination under the high power objective reveals a variable number of sperm per high power field, and a general average or range should be recorded. Motility characteristics should be noted, as well as evidence of poor morphology, agglutination, or in-place shaking movements.

Interpretation: There is no one normal finding. Each physician should have a concept of normality from repeated examination of multiple mucus samples. For instance, if most samples are examined 12 hours after intercourse, 8-12 sperm per high power field may be seen. Not only motility, but progressive forward movement is essential for a normal PCT.

3. If the PCT is abnormal:

> A. Verify that the mucus was evaluated at the right time in the cycle, just preovulatory.
> B. Confirm this subsequently by observing when the temperature rose by basal temperature chart (BTC) in that cycle.
> C. Ask when intercourse occurred.
> D. Verify that vaginal lubricants (K-Y jelly, vaseline, douches, and creams) were not used.
> E. Be sure that vaginal pool contamination was not sucked into the syringe, and that the cervix was wiped before aspiration.
> F. Identify specific causes of vaginitis, and treat these; Monilia, Trichomonas, Gardenella and other identifiable entities can cause an abnormal PCT.
> G. Repeat the PCT in another cycle to confirm persistent abnormality.

4. Proceed to:

A. Artificial insemination with husbands' specimen (AIH)

Technique: Inseminate with fresh ejaculate directly into cervical mucus or use cup insemination; examine mucus 2-6 hours later as for PCT

B. In vitro sperm-cervical mucus contact test (SCMCT or Kremer test)

Technique: Place drop of sperm contiguous to blob of mucus on glass side, __without__ cover slip, allow interface to form and examine under low power of microscope.

Interpretation: Sperm normally form phalanges and move rapidly into mucus, but the test is dependent upon the presence of good quality, nonviscous mucus.

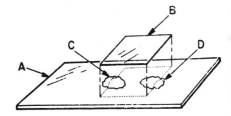

The SCMCT:

A) Microscope slide;
B) Cover slip;
C) Drop of semen;
D) Drop of cervical mucus;
E) Interphase between semen and cervical mucus;
F) Phalanx formation:
  The seminal plasma protruding into cervical mucus containing motile sperm.

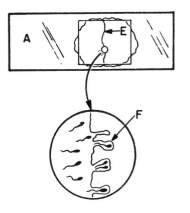

C. Sperm-cervical mucus cross-match testing.

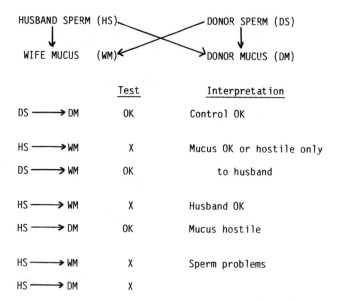

	Test	Interpretation
DS ⟶ DM	OK	Control OK
HS ⟶ WM	X	Mucus OK or hostile only
DS ⟶ WM	OK	to husband
HS ⟶ WM	X	Husband OK
HS ⟶ DM	OK	Mucus hostile
HS ⟶ WM	X	Sperm problems
HS ⟶ DM	X	

Donor mucus can be kept for about a week at room temperature, and slightly longer in the refrigerator. Alternatively, donor mucus can be frozen without destroying its usefulness. Obviously, it must be free of sperm. Patients undergoing ovulation induction with human menopausal gonadotropins (hMGs) or who are in an in vitro fertilization (IVF) cycle are good sources of estrogenized, profuse, watery cervical mucus, if they have had several days of abstinence.

D. Flat capillary tube penetration tests

1. The capillary tube may contain
        wife's mucus
        donor mucus
        bovine mucus (commercially available)
        synthetic mucus (investigational only)

2. The sperm can be
        husband
        donor

Front and lateral views of Kremer chambers and flat cylindrical capillary tubes used to study mucus penetrability by sperm.

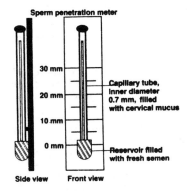

5. If no sperm in the PCT, and
   sperm are found after AIH, consider:

   A. Coital difficulties
         anatomic abnormalities (hypospadias, anteriorly
            displaced cervix)
         obesity
         impotence
         premature or failed ejaculation
   B. Use of spermicidal creams or jellies
   C. Vaginal lubricants

6. Performance Tests

The "performance tests," including sperm-cervical mucus penetration tests and cross-match testing should permit identification of:

   A. cervical mucus abnormalities
   B. semen abnormalities (see Male Factor, Chapter 13)
   C. specific sperm-mucus incompatibility

A. CERVICAL MUCUS ABNORMALITIES

Infected mucus should be obvious, but can only be diagnosed if the mucus is evaluated at the appropriate time in the cycle. It may be necessary to evaluate a patient's mucus every other day in conjunction with the BTC, to establish that the mucus is abnormal. Cellularity is normal just after menses and in the midluteal phase, and white cells observed at these times do not necessarily indicate infection.

Mycoplasma may be cultured from the cervical mucus of both infertile and fertile women. The significance of this finding is therefore unclear. Declomycin or tetracycline for 10 days is curative for this infection.

Treatment of infected mucus with a 10-day course of a broad spectrum antibiotic administered from the onset of menses is usually effective. Vibramycin, 100 mg daily, is an acceptable therapy.

Inadequate cervical mucus at an appropriate time in the cycle may be due to surgical treatment such as conization, or to cryosurgery or hot cautery therapy, with removal or destruction of the mucus-producing endocervical glands; or to a hormonal cause, with inadequate E_2 stimulation or an inability of the glands to respond to estrogen.

Treatment of inadequate mucus is usually unsatisfactory. Little can be done for destroyed glands, except to bypass them using intrauterine insemination. The administration of low-dose ethinyl estradiol, 10 ug, DES, 0.1 mg, or conjugated estrogens, 0.325 mg a day continually from cycle days 3-12 may be tried; ovulation will rarely be delayed. Basal temperature should be recorded and a repeat PCT obtained under treatment. The local administration of estrogen creams may be beneficial in the stubborn case, but, as estrogen is readily absorbed through the vaginal mucosa, care must be taken not to achieve circulating estrogen levels sufficient to inhibit ovulation. A brief but high dose of estrogen may also benefit the inadequate mucus. Ethinyl estradiol 100-200 ug daily for days 10-12 of the cycle, may improve mucus without inhibiting ovulation, but is likely to cause significant nausea.

Thick, viscous cervical mucus may respond to estrogen administration although a more fruitful approach is to explore why estrogen stimulation is lacking. Such drugs as guaifenesin (in Robitussin), potassium iodine and Alevaire are unlikely to produce much benefit.

Hostile mucus. Cervical mucus which appears to be uninfected and abundant, but which does not support sperm motility or penetration, must be further evaluated. A sperm mucus cross-match previously described is very useful in this setting. Donor semen, estrogenic donor mucus, wife's mucus, and husband's sperm are obtained, and both semen samples are run separately against the donor mucus, to ascertain if the husband's sperm show good progressive motility and viability within the donor mucus. Both semen samples are run against the wife's mucus as well. Thus, one can ascertain if the factor producing sperm immobility is a feature of the sperm sample, or of the wife's mucus.

A good quality mucus which does not support sperm survival should be checked with pH paper. Acidic cervical mucus may be treated with bicarbonate douches but considering that mucus and water are immiscible liquids, this treatment is probably empiric.

B. Antisperm Antibody (AsAb) Testing in the Female

A clue to the presence of antisperm antibodies (AsAb) is the observation of good quality mucus in which sperm are present but do not exhibit progressive motility; sperm can be seen to be "shaking" in place. Further evaluation should include:

1. Sperm Agglutination Testing: performed on male serum, female serum, and cervical mucus.

   A. Microscopic test: Franklin-Dukes Tray agglutination test (TAT)
   B. Macroscopic test: Kibrick gel agglutination test (GAT)
      Positive test: titer of 1:16 or greater

2. Sperm Immobilization testing: on male serum and female serum and cervical mucus

   A. Isojima, complement-dependent IgG or IgM
      Positive test: sperm immobilization value (SIV) 3.0 or greater

3. Other immunologic tests available in some centers include:

   A. Mixed antiglobulin reaction (MAR) IgG, IgA; done on semen only
   B. Immunobead binding
   C. Radiolabeled antiglobulin assay
   D. Enzyme-linked immunosorbent assay (ELISA)
   E. Spermocytotoxicity testing

Immunologic tests performed only on serum may not reflect antisperm activity locally, in the cervical mucus or higher in the reproductive tract. Cervical mucus must be specially prepared for testing, using Bromelin or other substances to put it into solution. Secretory IgA will <u>only</u> be present in the reproductive tract. IgM molecules are so large that they may not transude into the female tract from the serum, giving misleading serum results.

<u>Treatment</u> for AsAb in the female is usually unsatisfactory and there is no consensus as to approach. Condom contraception for 6 months followed by limited midcycle exposure has been recommended. High-dose corticosteroid treatment, for example, methylprednisolone (Medrol) 32 mg TID, from cycle day 21 for 10 days, is without documented efficacy; a significant complication of high-dose steroid treatment in both male and female is aseptic necrosis of the hip, which may occur well after treatment has been discontinued.

Intrauterine insemination has its advocates as has sperm washing and other techniques, but none has proven usefulness. The therapy is controversial, and side effects may be serious.

SUGGESTED READING

Blasco L: Clinical approach to the evaluation of sperm-cervical mucus interactions. Fertil Steril 28:1133, 1977.

Bronson RA, Cooper GW, Rosenfeld DL: Autoimmunity to spermatozoa: effect on sperm penetration of cervical mucus as reflected by postcoital testing. Fertil Steril 41:609, 1984.

Bronson R, Cooper G, Rosenfeld DL: Sperm antibodies: their role in infertility. Fertil Steril 42:171, 1984.

Fordney-Settlage D: A review of cervical mucus and sperm interactions in humans. Int J Fertil 26:161, 1981.

Katz DF, Overstreet JW, Tom RA, Hanson FW: Factors influencing the penetration of human spermatozoa into cervical mucus in vitro. Gamete Res 9:167, 1984.

Mathur S, Williamson HO, Baker ME, Rust PF, Holtz GL, Fudenberg HH: Sperm motility on postcoital testing correlates with male autoimmunity to sperm. Fertil Steril 41:81, 1984.

Mills RN, Katz DF: A flat capillary tube system for assessment of sperm movement in cervical mucus. Fertil Steril 29:43, 1978.

Chapter 15

The Uterine/Endometrial Factor

Anne Colston Wentz, M.D.

The uterine factor includes two types of uterine abnormalities which can cause infertility: (1) an anatomic abnormality, and (2) an endometrial factor, which constitutes a local intrauterine cause of implantation failure.

1. ANATOMIC UTERINE FACTOR

      A. Intrauterine Adhesions
      B. Leiomyomata
      C. Congenital Anomalies

2. ENDOMETRIAL UTERINE FACTOR

      A. Endometrial inadequacy without progesterone output deficiency
      B. Endometrial inadequacy with progesterone output deficiency

1. ANATOMIC UTERINE FACTOR

      A. Intrauterine Adhesions

Definition: Intrauterine adhesions (endometrial sclerosis, Asherman's syndrome) refers to the partial or complete obliteration of the uterine cavity by adherence of the uterine walls.

Incidence: The overall incidence of intrauterine adhesions is unknown, as diagnosis depends upon hysterosalpingography. The frequency of detection in the population of infertile women ranges from 5-39%.

Etiology: Uterine adhesion formation is usually related to postpartum or postabortal manipulation of the uterine cavity, particularly in the presence of infection. The most severe and extensive cases of intrauterine adhesions occur in relatively hypoestrogenic conditions requiring D & C, in which regeneration of endometrial tissue is inadequate. A protective effect of postpartum curettage appears to exist in the first 48 hours postpartum, and after 6 weeks; a higher incidence of intrauterine adhesion formation is diagnosed when curettage is performed in the interim.

Diagnosis: Intrauterine adhesions are initially found during routine hysterosalpingography performed during the basic infertility evaluation. Use of a short cannula is usually recommended if adhesions are suspected; however, if cervical or isthmic adhesions are present, the cannula must puncture or perforate these to distinguish between complete obliteration of the uterine cavity and intracervical scarring. Usually, adhesions are asymptomatic and unsuspected although occasionally associated with hypomenorrhea. Intrauterine adhesions are classified as mild, moderate or severe, based on the extent of cavity involved, the type of adhesions, and the menstrual pattern.

American Fertility Society Classification of Intrauterine Adhesions

Extent of Cavity Involved	< 1/3 1	1/3-2/3 2	> 2/3 4
Type of Adhesions	Filmy 1	Filmy & Dense 2	Dense 4
Menstrual Pattern	Normal 0	Hypomenorrhea 2	Amenorrhea 4

Prognosis for conception is dependent upon tubal patency.

	HSG SCORE	HYSTEROSCOPY SCORE
Stage I (Mild) - 1-4		
Stage II (Moderate) - 5-8	____	____
Stage III (Severe) - 9-12	____	____

Treatment: Treatment consists of lysis of intrauterine adhesions at D & C preferably under direct visualization with the hysteroscope. Thick adhesions may require incision with "hysteroscopic scissors" while delicate adhesions may be ruptured simply by the instillation of 32% Dextran-70. Alternatively, adhesions may be broken up using Hegar dilators.

A mechanical means of maintaining separation of the anterior and posterior walls of the uterine cavity following curettage is helpful; this may be accomplished using a Foley catheter with the bulb inflated to 5 cc, which is usually expelled in several days, or a 10F pediatric Foley catheter with a 3 cc bulb which may be retained for up to a week. The previous recommendation for IUD insertion is no longer an option.

Adjuvant therapy with estrogens and antibiotics is recommended. Conjugated estrogens, 2.5 mg BID for 30 to 60 days, followed by medroxyprogesterone acetate, 10 mg daily for 10 days, is an adequate course. Doxycycline, 50 mg BID for 10 days, is routinely used although the literature does not indicate a proven benefit of antibiotic coverage.

Follow-up hysterography is important, as recurrence is frequent. Although most patients will regain relatively normal menstrual patterns following lysis of intrauterine adhesions, nevertheless, the obstetrical results are less than entirely satisfactory. Early pregnancy wastage, as well as premature delivery, placenta accreta, and placenta percreta have been reported.

B. Leiomyomata ("Fibroids")

Leiomyomata are the most common pelvic tumors in women, although the exact incidence is unknown. Perhaps 20% of all women over age 30 years have myomata. These are ordinarily found on hysterosalpingography, or on routine pelvic examinations, and menorrhagia may result. Myomata do not usually cause infertility but interfere with implantation, and with pregnancy maintenance.

Patients with a myomatous uterus of 12 weeks' size or less may be observed for the occurrence of pregnancy for 6-12 months after diagnosis. Myomata of this size are infrequently associated with infertility and live birth is likely. Increasing uterine size, menorrhagia, fetal wastage or a distorted intrauterine cavity are all indications for surgical intervention.

For patients with larger myomata, treatment ordinarily consists of myomectomy, although various hormonal means of decreasing the size of myomata have been attempted. The myomectomy should be accomplished through a vertical midline uterine incision, which will reduce blood loss by restricting the incision to the least vascular area of the uterus; however the larger and more numerous the tumors, the greater the difficulty in removing them through a single anterior vertical incision. The same principle of using vertical incisions, kept as small and midline as possible, should be followed for 2nd, 3rd, and 4th incisions. A large submucous myoma which distorts the uterine cavity should be removed. The hysteroscope, or the urologic resectoscope, can be employed to remove submucous and pedunculated myomata up to 2-3 cm in size.

C. Congenital Anomalies

Uterine anomalies are frequently unrecognized because they are not associated with early pregnancy wastage. Most arcuate and septate uteri are not associated with miscarriage, although pregnancy wastage is increased overall in patients who have uterine anomalies. About 25% of these women will have problems with pregnancy loss, though second trimester pregnancy wastage is more common than early loss.

Surgical treatment of the septate uterus results in an 80% chance of live birth, although treatment with progesterone supplementation has proven beneficial, resulting in a 60% chance of delivery in patients having early pregnancy wastage. Surgical metroplasty may not be required in all patients, particularly in those with early loss who may benefit from progesterone administration. Most surgical resections for septate uteri can be accomplished transcervically using the hysteroscope, monitored by concomitant laparoscopy. Many technical approaches have been successful, including the urologic electrocautery, resectoscope, scissors, and laser vaporization.

Hysteroscopic management: Operative hysteroscopic incision of uterine septa, performed in conjunction with laparoscopy, is a safe and effective modality for treatment. Hysteroscopy is an outpatient procedure, avoids abdominal and uterine incisions, requires no long-term post-operative delay at attempting pregnancy, does not require cesarean section at subsequent pregnancy, is less expensive in terms of both time and money, and has less morbidity. Incision of the septum can be accomplished using hysteroscopic scissors, or, by substituting a urologic cystoscope for the hysteroscope, by resectoscope, and/or with electrocautery. Because of the relative avascularity of the septum, bleeding is usually minimal. Postoperative adjunctive therapy includes IUD or 16 Foley catheter insertion, the use of antibiotics, and treatment with estrogen followed by a progestational agent. Reproductive outcome is significantly improved, with approximately 70% of patients having a full-term delivery.

D. Endometritis

Endometritis is an unlikely cause of infertility or pregnancy wastage. However, abortion has been reported in patients diagnosed to have t-mycoplasma infection. Rarely, the finding of foci of lymphocytes read on endometrial biopsy may suggest treatment of an infertile patient with a broad spectrum antibiotic. It is otherwise difficult to attribute infertility to endometritis.

2. ENDOMETRIAL FACTOR

A. Luteal Phase Inadequacy without Progesterone Inadequacy

   1. First cycle after stopping Danazol
   2. Septate uterus
   3. Progesterone receptor defect
   4. ? Asherman's syndrome
   5. ? Infectious diseases

B. Luteal Phase Inadequacy with Progesterone Inadequacy

   1. Central etiology
   2. Metabolic etiology
   3. Gonadal etiology

A. Luteal Inadequacy without Progesterone Inadequacy

Etiology: Endometrial inadequacy without a documented defect in progesterone output can only be made by endometrial biopsy.

In the first cycle after stopping danazol, the endometrium is unlikely to be adequately stimulated, particularly if danazol has been administered at high dose for long duration. Inadequate placentation may be induced, which theoretically may result in second trimester abortion, or perhaps intrauterine growth retardation. For this reason, several investigators have advised using barrier contraception in the first cycle after stopping danazol; others have found no increase in abortion in patients achieving pregnancy in the first cycle after stopping danazol.

The septate uterus may have an inadequate vascular supply to the endometrium overlying the septum. Although this has never been studied in a controlled fashion, progesterone suppository administration (not surgical treatment) in patients with early miscarriage who had a septate uterus resulted in a 60% live birth rate.

The theoretical possibility of a progesterone receptor defect has been described; a progesterone receptor defect must be rare, but might be induced by an inadequate estrogen milieu or inadequate estrogen receptor synthesis.

Patients with Asherman's syndrome, or endometrial sclerosis, may have sufficient scarring to result in inadequate endometrial development when corpus luteum function is normal. Also unproven, the possibility that an infectious process, for example, Mycoplasma or Chlamydia infection, might be responsible for a deranged endometrial development.

Although rare, these entities would be completely missed if progesterone levels alone were used to make the diagnosis of luteal phase inadequacy, and if the endometrial biopsy were not employed.

B. Luteal Inadequacy with Progesterone Inadequacy

Etiology: The pathogenesis of luteal phase inadequacy is multifaceted. Inadequate folliculogenesis can clearly induce inadequate corpus luteum function. An adequate pool of primordial follicles is essential to follicular development. Hormonal inadequacy, including gonadotropin and steroid defects, as well as insufficiency of receptor site synthesis, all occurring before ovulation, may all result in disordered corpus luteum function. Metabolic defects in liver or kidney function, or defects in oxygenation can result in inappropriate enzyme and hormone synthesis. Luteal phase inadequacy can result from any defect of folliculogenesis.

Clearly, in many cases of endometrial inadequacy, there is a progesterone output deficiency or an abnormal progesterone to estradiol output ratio. However, making this diagnosis is very difficult, because of the variability of sex steroid output and the failure of a single sample to reflect corpus luteum function.

C. Diagnosis of Luteal Inadequacy

Diagnosis of luteal phase inadequacy by measurement of serum hormone levels is misleading and inconsistent because of the pulsatile nature of LH and progesterone output during the luteal phase. Serial progesterone measurements reflecting total luteal output of progesterone have been used to show that the area under the progesterone curve is less in patients with defective function of the corpus luteum than in normal controls; clearly, however, this approach to diagnosis is clinically impractical. Pooling of 3 blood samples taken 3 days apart in the midluteal phase also does not provide documentation of normal or abnormal luteal function or endometrial response. A single progesterone value is clearly of no assistance in establishing a diagnosis.

Daily samples for progesterone were obtained in 26 women who did not have endometrial inadequacy and in 10 women who did have an out-of-phase biopsy. Although the area under the progesterone output curve is less for those with a luteal phase endometrial defect, there is no difference between peak progesterone levels, or between samples on particular days during the luteal phase. Therefore, a single (or even several) blood samples taken for progesterone assay will not adequately reflect the effect of the corpus luteum steroid output on the endometrium.

Endometrial biopsy is the most reproducible diagnostic method, and although not quantitative, does indicate the pattern of hormone influence on the endometrial implantation site. The endometrial biopsy reading can be thought of as a bioassay of progesterone and estradiol effect at the endometrial level. The histologic pattern should reflect an adequate output of progesterone, and an appropriate ratio of progesterone to estradiol, if the expected secretory date coincides with the observed date.

In situations of endometrial inadequacy associated with normal progesterone output, the endometrial biopsy represents the only way to diagnose an inappropriately developed implantation site.

Technique: The appointment should be made premenstrually, preferably in relation to BTC chart elevation, and ideally on the 27th day of a 28-day cycle (or 1-2 days before expected menses).

1. The patient is placed in the lithotomy position, and examined to determine uterine position; the speculum is inserted, and the cervix visualized.
2. A small amount of Betadine is used to cleanse the region of the cervix and the external os.
3. Local anesthetic agent may be applied to the anterior lip; we use dental xylocaine.
4. The anterior lip of the cervix is grasped with a single-toothed tenaculum.
5. The uterus may be sounded, but this is not essential if a prior examination for uterine position has been performed.

6. The Novak curette is introduced into the endocervical canal, allowed to clear the internal os, and is then pushed to the fundus.
7. The curette is then turned such that either the anterior or posterior wall may be biopsied.
8. The biopsy is taken by a firm and rapid scraping of the curette down the wall of the uterus.
9. The piece of tissue is then blown out onto a paper towel (not a gauze square as it sticks) and examined. It should measure at least 2 cm in length, and be cylindrical.
10. The tissue must be immediately fixed as autolysis can occur rapidly; formalin is an appropriate fixative.
11. A tampon is placed in the vagina to tamponade cervical bleeding after the tenaculum is removed. The patient must be reminded to remove the tampon in 2 hours.
12. The patient should be reassured that some cramping is inevitable and that the discomfort is transient.

Interpretation: The biopsy is evaluated by the histologic criteria of Noyes, Hertig, and Rock and the histologic dating of the biopsy is recorded. The biopsy cannot be interpreted in relation to the patient's cycle until the date of her next menstrual period is known. At this time, the temperature chart is reviewed, and the presumed day of ovulation defined as day 14. The day of onset of menses is arbitrarily called day 28. All three dates, the histologic, the day postovulation, and the day premenses should coincide.

Because a biopsy taken 2 days before the onset of the next period should appear similar in all women, the time of the next period is then the reference date and the patient is instructed to report the first day of her next menstrual period so that the biopsy can be interpreted. Since day 28 has been assigned as the day of menstruation; a biopsy obtained 2 days before the menses should have the appearance of secretory day 26 endometrium.

To make the diagnosis, the biopsy date must be out-of-phase by 2 days or more from the expected date as judged from the next menstrual period; for example, read secretory day 23-24 on ideal day 26. Thus, the dating of the endometrium depends on the onset of the next menstrual period, and the diagnosis and dating are both unrelated to the onset of the previous menstrual period and, for all practical purposes, the time of ovulation, which is impossible to judge accurately.

199

To be significant, the biopsy must be out-of-phase by 2 or more days in at least 2 cycles.

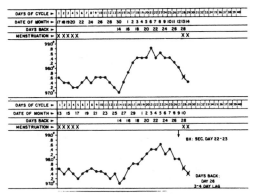

<u>Top.</u> A 28-day menstrual cycle with a luteal span of 14 days may not have adequate progesterone support. <u>Middle.</u> A biopsy (BX) taken on cycle day 26 was diagnosed to show a histologic pattern typical of secretory day 22-23. The next menstrual period came 2 days following the biopsy. Assigning day 28 to the day of onset of menses, a biopsy taken 2 days before should have been diagnosed as secretory day 26. The endometrial pattern, therefore, is out of phase by at least 3-4 days.

For the proper diagnosis of luteal phase inadequacy, the endometrial biopsy must be properly taken, and obtained within 1-2 days of the expected menstrual period, as calculated by temperature charts, history, or knowledge of when ovulation occurred. A biopsy taken after the onset of menstrual bleeding is too disrupted to date accurately, since the degree of leukocytic infiltration and decidual response under the capsule determines the date after ideal secretory day 25. Because the capsule is disrupted and shed in the earlier phases of menstruation, a biopsy taken after the onset of bleeding is usually inadequate. A biopsy taken at the time of implantation, approximately day 21 or 22 of the ideal menstrual cycle, barely reflects the progesterone output from the corpus luteum because the endometrium has only been exposed to a maximum of 7 days of progesterone output. If the endometrial biopsy is to be used as a bioassay of progesterone output, it should be taken as close as possible to the expected menses to reflect the entire luteal activity. Although the endometrial pattern at the time of implantation is probably important, progesterone apparently has other effects necessary for maintenance of an early pregnancy. Thus, it is the total progesterone output in which we are interested.

Summary: 1. Take biopsy within 2 days of menstruation
           2. Assign "day 28" to day of menstruation
           3. Count back to day of biopsy
           4. Ascertain if in- or out-of-phase

Examples: bx Aug 5, read as secretory day 26
           NMP Aug 7 = day 28
           bx on Aug 5 should be day 26, is day 26, so therefore
                is in phase

           bx Aug 5, read as secretory day 22
           NMP Aug 7 = day 28
           bx on Aug 5 should be day 26, is day 22, therefore is
                4 days out-of-phase

D. High-Risk Population

Since the etiology may be elusive, it makes more sense to concentrate attention on those patients with a higher likelihood of having luteal phase inadequacy, and to making the diagnosis in these patients. These include patients who:

1) have recurrent early pregnancy wastage
2) are receiving clomiphene citrate for ovulation induction
3) have hyperprolactinemia
4) are undergoing strenuous athletic conditioning (running, ballet, gymnastics)
5) have unexplained infertility
6) have endometriosis
7) are in the first 1-2 cycles after an abortion, delivery or stopping oral contraceptives
8) are over the age of 35 years

In the office setting, these patients would be considered to be at risk, and the diagnosis of luteal phase inadequacy should be actively sought.

Some reports suggest that as many as 30% of biopsies may be out-of-phase; however, the defect must be repetitive to be significant and overall, no more than perhaps 5% of women will be diagnosed as having a repetitive, clinically significant defect. If the biopsy sampling is limited to those at greater risk, obviously the incidence will increase.

E. Treatment of Luteal Phase Inadequacy

The presence of a defect can be established, but the hormonal etiology is not usually diagnosed; however, approaches to therapy are straightforward, involving either stimulation of luteal function or substitution for the deficiency. Human chorionic gonadotropin (hCG) directly stimulates luteal activity; clomiphene citrate would indirectly improve luteal activity only if folliculogenesis were somehow bettered. Substitution therapy is accomplished using vaginal, rectal or intramuscular progesterone, but never using a progestational agent. Theoretically, if a luteal phase defect is due to an inadequate FSH increase before menstruation, then an increased dose of CC might correct the disorder. However, since this is a rarely diagnosed etiology, CC is not indicated in the initial therapy of a spontaneous luteal defect.

From a practical standpoint, substitution for the progesterone inadequacy with the administration of progesterone has proved most successful in the treatment of the inadequate luteal phase due to any of several etiologies. The choice of progesterone supplementation, however, is best reserved for those patients:

1) with normal follicular phase length
2) who have normal prolactin levels
3) have a normal hysterosalpingogram
4) who have no other clearly diagnosable cause of luteal phase inadequacy
5) who are 35 years of age or less

The endometrial development associated with an adequate progesterone output appears to be at least as important as the progesterone secretion. Therefore, since progesterone administration can be shown to induce a normal development of the endometrium, this has become our treatment of choice for properly selected patients.

For successful therapy of a luteal phase defect, an accurate basal temperature recording is essential for the proper timing of therapy. Preovulatory administration of progesterone may block ovulation, which is then misinterpreted as an early pregnancy. Successful therapy must be begun in the cycle in which ovulation related to the pregnancy occurs, because normal endometrial development is needed to allow normal implantation and the maintenance of an early pregnancy. Especially in patients with recurrent miscarriage, therapy begun after the missed menses is inadequate and does not reliably prevent implantation failure.

Substitution therapy using progesterone vaginal suppositories is our primary therapeutic approach because of its simplicity, lack of complications, and good results. The patient should begin substitution after at least three days of temperature rise (for most patients) above 97.8°F. Progesterone support must begin early enough to be therapeutic, and late enough not to interupt ovulation; the postovulatory temperature increase will not be masked or inhibited by progesterone administration after three days of rise. Therapy should be continued until menses, and ordinarily a delay in menstruation does not occur. An occasional patient will have an elevated temperature in the follicular part of her cycle, not dropping to low levels until shortly before ovulation; therefore, it is practical not to begin substitution therapy until after day 17 of the cycle, and then only after the basal temperature has risen.

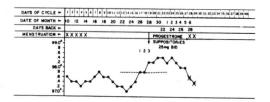

When this patient's temperature had been at or greater than 97.8°F for at least 3 consecutive days, ovulation has presumptively occurred and progesterone support should be begun. The suppositories are continued until the onset of the menses, and a repeat biopsy is indicated a day or two before the expected onset of menses to document correction of the endometrial defect.

Documentation of correction of the defect must be made by endometrial biopsy in the first or second treated cycle. At least 13% of patients will have a persistent defect despite treatment. If the defect persists, a higher progesterone dose or an alternative treatment approach may be required.

The significance of luteal phase inadequacy continues to be controversial. It is difficult to find a study with sufficient numbers of patients to prove statistically that the diagnosis and treatment of luteal phase inadequacy change the fertility potential of patients. The population studied by Daly does show enhanced fecundity in those patients with endometrial dysmaturity corrected by progesterone suppositories. Patients with recurrent fetal wastage found to have luteal inadequacy are clearly benefitted, and live-birth potential with progesterone treatment in these patients approaches statistical significance.

WHEN PREGNANCY OCCURS

Therapy is continued in the early stages of pregnancy, with documentation of a normal rise of βhCG; progesterone supplementation is discontinued when fetal heart motion is seen.

Some questions have risen as to the association of progesterone administration with congenital anomalies. Sufficient patients have been treated with progesterone to achieve statistical significance, and no increased incidence of congenital anomalies can be identified. The congenital anomaly rate in 293 control cases was 4.2% and in 155 progesterone treated cases was 4.5%; in another series, 1400 control patients were found to have 19 anomalies for a rate per thousand of 13.57; 837 treated cases had 12 congenital anomalies, for a rate of 14.34 per thousand. In other studies, congenital anomalies, particularly masculinization or ambiguity of the external genitalia, were associated with the use of the C-21 and 19-nortestosterone compounds in early pregnancy, but there was no increased incidence of anomalies with the use of natural progesterone or hydroxyprogesterone. The continuation of progesterone suppositories until about 10 weeks' gestational age, or fetal heart on ultrasound is important in the management of any patient documented to have luteal phase insufficiency who achieves early pregnancy taking progesterone substitution therapy.

204

SUGGESTED READING

Bergquist CA, Rock JA, Jones HW Jr: Pregnancy outcome following treatment of intrauterine adhesions. Int J Fertil 26:107, 1981.

Breen JL, Neubecker R, Gregori CA, Franklin JE Jr: Placenta accreta, increta, and percreta. A survey of 40 cases. Obstet Gynecol 49:43, 1977.

Buttram VC Jr, Reiter RC: Uterine leiomyomata: Etiology, symptomatology, and management. Fertil Steril 36:433, 1981.

Czernobilsky B: Endometritis and infertility. Fertil Steril 30:119, 1978.

Daly DC, Walters CA, Soto-Albors CE, Riddick DH: Endometrial biopsy during treatment of luteal phase defects is predictive of therapeutic outcome. Fertil Steril 40:305, 1983.

Greenwood SM, Moran JJ: Chronic endometritis: Morphologic and clinical observations. Obstet Gynecol 58:176, 1981.

Noyes RW, Hertig AT, Rock J: Dating the endometrial biopsy. Fertil Steril 1:3, 1950.

Schenker JG, Margalioth EJ: Intrauterine adhesions: an updated appraisal. Fertil Steril 37:593, 1982.

Wallach EE: The uterine factor in infertility. Fertil Steril 23:138, 1972.

Wentz AC: Progesterone therapy of the inadequate luteal phase, in Givens JR (ed): Clinical Use of Sex Steroids. Chicago, Year Book Medical Publishers, Inc., 1980.

Wentz AC, Herbert CM, Maxson WS, Garner CH: Outcome of progesterone treatment of luteal phase inadequacy. Fertil Steril 41:856, 1984.

Chapter 16

Tubal and Peritoneal Factor

Carl M. Herbert III, M.D.

PERITONEAL FACTOR

Approximately 25-50% of females whose evaluations have shown no explanation for infertility are found to have a peritoneal factor at the time of laparoscopy. Peritoneal factors are usually either (1) endometriosis or (2) pelvic adhesive disease. For a discussion of endometriosis see Chapter 18. Pelvic adhesions arise from damage or alteration of peritoneal surfaces causing abnormal agglutination of the serosal surfaces of bowel, uterus, fallopian tube and/or ovary.

Adhesion formation is thought to start with either inflammation (infection), foreign body reaction (talc or suture), or peritoneal trauma (surgery). These insults lead to mast cell release of vasoactive kinins and histamine causing an increase in capillary permeability followed by formation of a serosanguinous exudate and deposition of fibrin. If plasminogen activator and plasmin are subsequently released by adjacent tissue, fibrinolysis and clean healing occur. However, crush injury, tissue repair under tension, and/or edema lead to ischemia, suppression of plasminogen activator, and failure of fibrinolysis. The persistent fibrin forms a permanent adhesion which undergoes varying degrees of invasion by fibroblasts and capillaries. The differences in degree give rise to the two types of adhesions characterized clincally as (1) thin, filmy, avascular, allowing easy tissue repair and (2) thick, fibrous, organized, vascular, difficult to accomplish permanent tissue separation.

Factors causing the development of pelvic adhesions frequently are involved in creation of tubal damage. The major etiologies for adhesions and tubal disease are: infection, endometriosis, and surgery. Infection may take the form of ascending through the vagina, cervix, uterus, and tubes forming an endometritis and/or salpingitis picture. This condition is termed pelvic inflammatory disease (PID). The two most common etiologies are Neisseria gonorrhoeae and Chlamydia trachomatis. Factors which predispose to development of PID include multiple sexual partners, use of an intrauterine device (IUD), and instrumentation of the uterus. Modern antibiotics have decreased the mortality associated with pelvic infections. However, postinfectious infertility remains a problem. Multiple episodes of PID appear to cause progressive damage and infertility (Westrom, 1975).

Episodes of Acute PID	Tubal Occlusion Rates
1	12.8%
2	35.5%
3	75.0%

Appendicitis has also been shown to increase infertility especially if there is rupture of the appendix. Other inflammatory processes in the peritoneal cavity including diverticulitis, regional ileitis, and traumatic peritonitis can result in adhesion formation and infertility.

Any form of surgical intervention in the pelvis may lead to adhesion formation. Surgical procedures on the ovary are especially prone to adhesion formation. If at all possible, operations like excision of a hemorrhagic corpus luteum or ovarian wedge resection should be avoided.

With the advent of "microsurgical" techniques, improvement in prevention of iatrogenic infertility and improved pregnancy rates during infertility surgery have been achieved. These techniques basically include:

1. Atraumatic handling of tissue
2. Use of delicate instruments
3. Use of fine nonreactive suture
4. Use of magnification (loopes or microscope).

Diagnosis of pelvic adhesive disease is best made visually during laparoscopy. This procedure is an important part of all infertility evaluations and provides both diagnostic and therapeutic potential. Laparoscopy is done as an outpatient procedure and offers the opportunity to perform operations previously requiring laparotomy (i.e., adhesiolysis, treatment of endometriosis, and salpingostomy). Small instruments with unipolar or bipolar cautery capability and more recently lasers are utilized through the laparoscope to accomplish surgical intervention. Types of lasers that have been utilized effectively through the laparoscope include CO_2, Argon, Nd:YAG, and KTP.

Prevention of adhesion formation or reformation is an important part of fertility surgery. A number of. different types of medications have been employed.

Antiadhesion Medications

Class	Agents	Mechanism of Action
Antibiotic	Doxycycline (Vibramycin)	Prevent infection
Glucocorticoid	Dexamethasone (Decadron)	Anti-inflammatory, Stabilize mast cells,
Antihistamine	Promethazine (Phenergan)	Prevent serosanguinous exudate formation
Nonsteroidal Anti-Inflammatory	Ibuprofen (Motrin)	Anti-prostaglandin

Other substances such as high molecular weight dextran (Hyskon, 32% dextran 70) or carboxymethyl cellulose have been used to prevent peritoneal surfaces from adhering to one another. The true efficacy of any of these adjuncts has not been definitively proven. Neveretheless, prevention of tissue desiccation during surgery using frequent irrigation with lactated Ringer's solution with heparin (5000 units/liter) is recommended. When appropriate, the omentum should be removed or tacked into the upper abdomen to prevent pelvic involvement.

TUBAL FACTOR

Tubal factor is found to be at least part of the etiology for infertility in 30-50% of infertile women. Diagnosis of the tubal factor should involve the use of both laparoscopy and hysterosalpingography. These procedures should be considered complimentary as each has its own rate of false-positives and false-negatives, especially for tubal patency testing.

The hysterosalpingogram (HSG) provides evaluation of the endometrial cavity (submucus fibroids, endometrial polyps); evaluation of the interstitial portion of the tube (salpingitis isthmica nodosa, tubal polyps); and evaluation of the distal tubal lumen (intraluminal synechiae, point of tubal occlusion). These data are not available through laparoscopy alone. A Rubin's test (insufflation of CO_2) is inaccurate for fertility assessment and should no longer be used. Performance of the HSG should occur during the proliferative phase of the menstrual cycle after cessation of menses and before ovulation. Selection of contrast media for performance of an HSG remains somewhat controversial.

Overall, there appears to be an increased pregnancy rate for 3-4 months after an HSG in some infertile couples. This increased pregnancy rate is reported to be 1 to 2 times greater when using oil-based rather than water-based contrast media. However, water-based contrast media provides better tubal mucosal detail and more rapid absorption especially if nonpatent hydrosalpinges are encountered. Some authors have recommended the use of water contrast media followed by 3-5 cc of oil contrast media if normal patent tubes are encountered. Individuals found to have tubal disease at HSG should receive prophylactic antibiotics afterward (doxycycline, 100 mg PO BID for 5 days). Individuals known to have tubal disease should receive prophylactic antibiotics both before and after their procedure.

Treatment

Treatment of tubal factor infertility has traditionally been surgical. The surgical techniques vary with the region of the tube that is involved.

Fimbrial agglutination with maintenance of tubal patency can occur at the distal end of the tube. Management of fimbrial agglutination can be done either laparoscopically or at laparotomy. Adhesiolysis of the fimbrial bands is accomplished with microtip cautery or laser vaporization. In most cases, lysis of one or more bands will allow reasonably normal fimbria to expand adequately but occasionally one or more fine sutures (8-0) is needed to ensure adequate patency. Ovarian adhesiolysis is often needed in conjunction with fimbrioplasty procedures. Success rates after fimbrioplasty/adhesiolysis procedures depend on the type of adhesions and degree of involvement but often pregnancy rates are reported $\geq 60\%$.

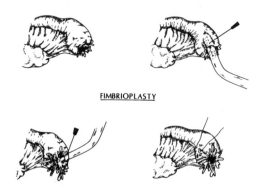

FIMBRIOPLASTY

Distal tubal occlusion, hydrosalpinx, is managed by performance of a neosalpingostomy. Cruciate incisions in the distal tube can be made with either microtip cautery or laser. The tubal flaps created by the incision are then either sewn back onto the tubal serosa or desiccated on the serosal surface with a defocused laser beam to maintain tubal patency. Fertility after this surgery is dependent on: (1) thickeness of the tubal wall, (2) degree of mucosal damage, and (3) degree of dilatation. Based on the severity of these factors, pregnancy rates have been quoted at 15-40%. This procedure can be performed laparoscopically but not usually as the primary repair attempt. Postoperative hydrotubation is no longer recommended.

NEOSALPINGOSTOMY

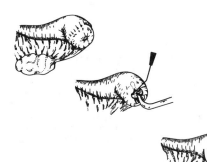

Midtubal occlusion is most often secondary to a sterilization procedure. Reversal of this sterilization requires resection of the occluded portion of tube with primary reanastomosis. Use of microsurgical techniques have significantly improved the success of this operation. Other factors affecting success include:

1. Type of sterilization (clip or fallope ring > Pomeroy partial salpingectomy > cautery > fimbriectomy)
2. Tubal length after reanastomosis (< 4 cm markedly reduces pregnancy rates)
3. Area of tube reanstomosed (equal-sized lumen reanastomoses are more successful with isthmic-isthmic providing the highest pregnancy rates).

Depending upon the above factors, pregnancy rates have been reported at 40-80% after sterilization reversal.

210

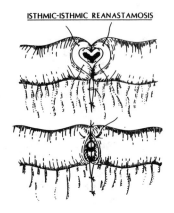

ISTHMIC-ISTHMIC REANASTAMOSIS

Surgically establishing tubal patency does not ensure a normal tube. All patients with tubal factor infertility are at an increased risk for an ectopic pregnancy. The majority of ectopic pregnancies occur in the ampullary portion of the fallopian tube. These may be managed conservatively via a linear salpingostomy either laparoscopically or during laparotomy; or if more advanced, radical therapy includes salpingectomy. Intrauterine pregnancy rates following conservative management of the ectopic pregnancy range 40-60% with repeat ectopic rates being 10-15%. If salpingectomy is necessary, conservation of the ipsilateral ovary is recommended.

SALPINGOSTOMY

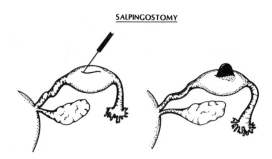

Proximal tubal or cornual occlusion usually involves postinfectious fibrosis or salpingitis isthmica nodosa. Repair involves resection of this damaged tissue and either a microsurgical reanastomosis or a tubal reimplantation procedure. Postoperative pregnancy rates are higher with a reanastomosis (40-60%) than with reimplantation (15-40%) and caesarean section is recommended for patients who conceive after a reimplantation procedure.

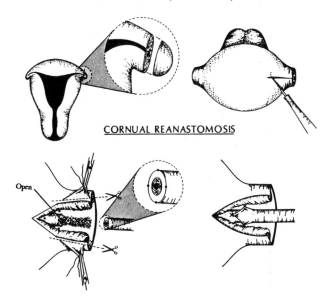

CORNUAL REANASTOMOSIS

Pregnancy rates after repair of tubes with both proximal and distal damage (bipolar tubal disease) are less than 10%. Similarly, pregnancy rates after repeat tubal surgery for failure of the initial procedure are less than 20% with a significant risk for ectopic pregnancy. For these patients and those with severe pelvic adhesive disease, in vitro fertilization/embryo transfer (IVF/ET) is the treatment of choice. The pregnancy rates for patients reaching the stage of embryo transfer are approximately 20-25% at present. If and when IVF/ET achieves a pregnancy rate > 50%, many of the indications for difficult tubal surgery will disappear. This is especially true since the development of nonoperative ultrasound guided technologies for aspiration of oocytes (see Chapter 21).

SUGGESTED READING

Buttram VC Jr, Reiter RC: Surgical Treatment of the Infertile Female. Baltimore, Williams & Wilkins, 1985.

DeCherney AH, Polan ML: In Ryan JD Jr (ed): Reproductive Surgery. Chicago, Year Book Medical Publishers, Inc., 1987.

Gomel V: Microsurgery in Female Infertility. Boston, Little, Brown and Company, 1983.

Jones HW Jr, Rock JA: Reparative and Constructive Surgery of the Female Generative Tract. Baltimore, Williams & Wilkins, 1983.

Speroff L: Seminars in Reproductive Endocrinology. New York, Thieme-Stratton Inc, 1984.

Westrom L: Effect of acute pelvic inflammatory disease on infertility. Am J Obstet Gynecol 121:707-713, 1975.

Winfield AC, Wentz AC: Diagnostic Imaging of Infertility. Baltimore, Williams & Wilkins, 1987.

Chapter 17

Endometriosis

Carl M. Herbert III, M.D.

DEFINITION

Endometriosis denotes the presence of functioning ectopic
endometrial tissue, including both glands and stroma, located
outside the uterine cavity. Adenomyosis (internal endometriosis)
defines endometrium found within the myometrium and is considered a
separate clinical entity. Endometriosis is most frequently found
within the female pelvis, however, it can be found at such distant
sites as brain, lung, pericardium, and appendix and has been
described in males. An individual endometriosis lesion is termed an
implant. Implants can vary in size and degree of subperitoneal
invasion. Palpable implants are termed nodules. Implants on the
ovary which become cystic and contain hemosiderin material are
termed endometriomas. Implants can produce an intense inflammatory
response which secondarily causes adhesion formation. The
therapeutic approach to management of endometriosis, therefore,
includes treatment of both primary implants and secondary adhesive
disease. Malignant transformation of endometriosis is so rare that
it should not be a consideration in the clinical management of most
patients. However, the coexistence of endometriosis and epithelial
ovarian malignancies, especially endometroid carcinoma, should be
remembered in any patient with ovarian enlargement, i.e.,
endometriomas.

EPIDEMIOLOGY

Endometriosis depends upon estrogen stimulation for growth and
propagation and has rarely been described before the menarche. The
exact incidence of endometriosis among women in the reproductive age
group has never been satisfactorily established. A best estimate
based on numerous studies would put the overall incidence at 5% or
less in the general population. Of women undergoing laparotomies
for gynecologic disease, 11-52% have been found to have
endometriosis. Among infertility patients, the prevalence of
endometriosis has been reported in the range of 40-50% and as high

as 75% among women who have undergone laparoscopy and in whom no other infertility factor has been identified. There is an increased incidence of endometriosis among women with mullerian anomalies and uterine outflow abnormalities. Endometriosis has been found in over 50% of teenagers who undergo laparoscopy for pelvic pain. The average age of diagnosis for endometriosis has decreased with the use of laparoscopy and now is in the range of 25-29 years. Recent studies do not show a correlation between the age at diagnosis and severity of endometriosis. Although there was once thought to be racial differences, recent studies show similar incidences in a variety of different racial groups. There is evidence, however, that a hereditary factor may be important for some populations. Inheritence patterns indicate a polygenic multifactorial mode of inheritence.

ETIOLOGIES

Numerous theories have been developed to explain the histogenesis of endometriosis. No one theory adequately explains the variety of clinical presentations which occur. The three major hypotheses are: (1) direct implantation (Sampson); (2) lymphatic/vascular dissemination (Halban); and (3) coelomic metaplasia (Meyers).

Direct Implantation: Studies have shown that retrograde regurgitation of blood and endometrial tissue occurs with menstrual flow in most women. These endometrial fragments may be viable and implant on various areas in the pelvis. They subsequently cycle under the influence of steroid hormones similar to the normal endometrium within the uterus. Animal models which obstruct the normal menstrual effluent and produce transtubal retrograde menstruation can create endometriosis. Similarly, abnormalities in the human such as imperforate hymen, transverse vaginal septum, cervical atresia, or severe cervical stenosis are frequently found in association with endometriosis. Endometrial fragments which are transplanted purposefully in animal models or iatrogenically during closing of episiotomy or caesarean section incisions postpartum can survive and cause cyclic symptomatology.

Decreased immune surveillance has been proposed as an explanation for implantation and survival of ectopic endometrial fragments. Preliminary studies in both animals and humans indicate a deficit in the cell mediated immune response.

Lymphatic/Vascular Dissemination: Endometrial cells, similar to gynecologic malignancies, may be picked up by the lymphatic and blood supply and carried to distant locations in the body. This theory would help explain the presence of endometriosis in such distant organs as the brain, lung, kidney, pericardium, and thigh.

Coelomic Metaplasia: The germinal epithelium of the ovary, endoemtrium, and peritoneum all originate from the same coelomic epithelium. The coelomic cells are totipotent and are theorized to undergo metaplastic transformation under the influence of menstrual irritation and hormonal stimulation. This theory has been used to help explain the presence of endometriosis in females with primary amenorrhea and without functioning uterine endometrium as well as in males after prolonged treatment with estrogen.

CLINICAL SYMPTOMATOLOGY

The classic symptom triad for patients with endometriosis is dysmenorrhea, dyspareunia, and infertility. However, patients will present with a spectrum of symptoms ranging from asymptomatic to complete disability. There is poor correlation between the severity of painful symptoms and the severity of disease. Mild endometriosis may cause significantly disabling dysmenorrhea and dyspareunia while large endometriomas may be asymptomatic and diagnosed on an annual pelvic exam.

Dysmenorrhea: Endometriosis is the most common cause of secondary dysmenorrhea. The etiology of this dysmenorrhea may relate to direct peritoneal inflammation and irritation by implants and/or prostaglandin stimulation of myometrial hypercontractility. Dysmenorrhea secondary to endometriosis typically presents before the onset of menses, is progressive in nature, and only partially relieved by the administration of prostaglandin synthetase inhibitors or oral contraceptives. Endometriosis involvement of the rectovaginal septum or uterosacral ligaments may cause pain referred to the rectum or lower sacral regions and be associated with constipation and dyschesia.

Dyspareunia: Painful intercourse associated with endometriosis is typically described as deep penetration dyspareunia. This same pain is frequently reproducible on gynecologic bimanual examination. This pain may be secondary to stretching of pelvic peritoneal surfaces involved with endometrial implants; movement of pelvic structures adherent with pelvic adhesions; direct contact with a fixed retroverted uterus. Symptoms are frequently more severe perimenstrually.

Infertility: Between 20% and 66% of women with endometriosis will experience some degree of infertility. Approximately 25% of infertile patients with endometriosis are multigravidas. Postulated

216

mechanisms for infertility associated with endometriosis include the following:

A. Mechanical factors: Severe cases of endometriosis are associated with pelvic adhesions and scarring which can limit tubal mobility and distort the normal tubal-ovarian anatomy. Although salpingitis has been described in association with endometriosis, there is rarely fallopian tube obstruction in this condition. Mild cases of endometriosis rarely involve mechanical factors.

B. Prostaglandins: Increased prostaglandin levels in peritoneal fluid have been reported from women with endometriosis. Similarly, the breakdown products of thromboxane A-2 and prostacyclin have been found to be increased in the peritoneal fluid. Prostaglandins could adversely effect fertility by increasing tubal motility and altering ovum transport, producing a toxic effect on the early embryo, preventing implantation, and/or causing a luteolytic effect at the level of the ovary. However, a number of recent studies have been unable to demonstrate consistently increased prostanoid concentrations in peritoneal fluid.

C. Macrophage Activation: Increased numbers of mononuclear phagocytes have been found in the peritoneal and tubal fluid of infertility patients with endometriosis. These peritoneal macrophages demonstrate an enhanced ability to phagocytize spermatozoa. They may also disrupt normal fertilization and embryo development.

D. Luteinized Unruptured Follicle (LUF) Syndrome: LUF syndrome has been noted to occur more frequently in patients with endometrosis. However, the criteria for a diagnosis of LUF syndrome are not standarized and, therefore, this association must be considered speculative.

E. Luteal Phase Defect (LPD): Although ovulatory disturbances and luteal phase defects have been described in association with endometriosis, controlled studies comparing serum hormone levels and endometrial biopsies have failed to show consistent defects.

F. Spontaneous Abortions: Spontaneous abortions in infertility patients with endometriosis have been reported to occur in 10-49% of pregnancies. Some of the higher values may be due to patient selection bias. However, most studies demonstrate a decrease in spontaneous abortions after treatment.

Distal Disease: Endometriosis can involve organ systems distant from the pelvis. The hallmark of symptoms created by distal implants is cyclic catamenial exacerbations. The following is a list of organ systems and symptoms that occur only with menstruation; brain seizures, migraine headaches; lungs (pneumothorax), hemoptysis; urinary tract (hematuria, ureteral obstruction, dysuria); intestinal tract (constipation, hematochesia); skin (swollen bluish colored scar). All of these symptoms occur only at the time of menses with asymptomatic intervals between.

DIAGNOSIS

Physical Examination

A. Physical findings are suggestive but not diagnostic.

B. Bimanual examination findings may include:

1. General pelvic tenderness
2. "Shotty nodularity" or "cobblestones" on the uterosacral ligaments and in the posterior cul-de-sac.
3. Thickening of the rectovaginal septum
4. A retroflexed, "fixed" uterus
5. Enlarged, tender and/or "fixed" ovaries

Surgical Diagnosis

A. Definite diagnosis of endometriosis requires visualization of implants.

B. An outpatient double-puncture, laparoscopic approach with some form of intravaginal cervically attached uterine elevation is recommended to:

1. Avoid an unnecessary laparotomy.
2. Provide full mobilization of the uterus and both ovaries to inspect their undersurfaces and deep in the posterior cul-de-sac.
3. Allow full pelvic visualization by manipulation of the bowel and aspiration of peritoneal fluid.

218

   C. A comprehensive systematic routine during laparoscopy will
       ensure all peritoneal surfaces are observed and a diagnosis
       is not missed.

   D. As endometrial implants have a characteristic appearance,
       routine biopsy to confirm the diagnosis is not necessary.
       Atypical lesions suspicious for malignancy should be
       biopsied.

   E. Use of photography or video equipment is beneficial for
       photodocumentation and education purposes.

The diagram below shows the percentage of patients with
laparoscopically documented endometrial implants in various pelvic
locations. (Reproduced by permission from Olive DL, Haney AF:
Endometriosis. In DeCherney AH: Reproductive Failure, New York,
Churchill Livinstone, 1986.)

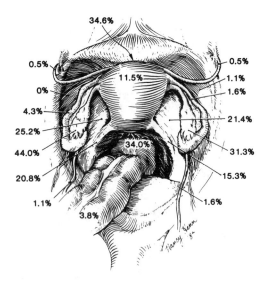

Anatomic locations
of endometriosis implants in
182 consecutive infertility patients found to have endometriosis by laparoscopy. The
rates shown indicate the percent of all patients with implants in a given locale.

THE AMERICAN FERTILITY SOCIETY
REVISED CLASSIFICATION OF ENDOMETRIOSIS

Patient's Name _____ Date _____

Stage I   (Minimal) - 1-5
Stage II (Mild)   - 6-15
Stage III (Moderate) - 16-40
Stage IV (Severe)   - >40
Total _____

Laparoscopy _____ Laparotomy _____ Photography _____
Recommended Treatment _____

Prognosis _____

PERITONEUM	ENDOMETRIOSIS	<1cm	1-3cm	>3cm
	Superficial	1	2	4
	Deep	2	4	6
OVARY	R Superficial	1	2	4
	Deep	4	16	20
	L Superficial	1	2	4
	Deep	4	16	20

	POSTERIOR CULDESAC OBLITERATION	Partial	Complete
		4	40

	ADHESIONS	<1/3 Enclosure	1/3-2/3 Enclosure	>2/3 Enclosure
OVARY	R Filmy	1	2	4
	Dense	4	8	16
	L Filmy	1	2	4
	Dense	4	8	16
TUBE	R Filmy	1	2	4
	Dense	4*	8*	16
	L Filmy	1	2	4
	Dense	4*	8*	16

*If the fimbriated end of the fallopian tube is completely enclosed, change the point assignment to 16.

Additional Endometriosis: _____ | Associated Pathology: _____

To Be Used with Normal Tubes and Ovaries
L   R

To Be Used with Abnormal Tubes and/or Ovaries
L   R

220

EXAMPLES & GUIDELINES

STAGE I (MINIMAL)	STAGE II (MILD)	STAGE III (MODERATE)

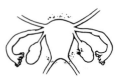

PERITONEUM
Superficial Endo   —   1-3cm   - 2
R. OVARY
Superficial Endo   —   < 1cm   - 1
Filmy Adhesions   —   < 1/3   - 1
       TOTAL POINTS   4

PERITONEUM
Deep Endo   —   > 3cm   - 6
R. OVARY
Superficial Endo   —   < 1cm   - 1
Filmy Adhesions   —   < 1/3   - 1
L. OVARY
Superficial Endo   —   < 1cm   - 1
       TOTAL POINTS   9

PERITONEUM
Deep Endo   —   > 3cm   - 6
CULDESAC
Partial Obliteration   - 4
L. OVARY
Deep Endo   —   1-3cm   - 16
       TOTAL POINTS   26

STAGE III (MODERATE)	STAGE IV (SEVERE)	STAGE IV (SEVERE)

 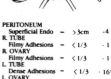 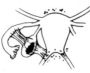 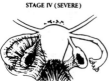

PERITONEUM
Superficial Endo   —   > 3cm   -4
R. TUBE
Filmy Adhesions   —   < 1/3   - 1
R. OVARY
Filmy Adhesions   —   < 1/3   - 1
L. TUBE
Dense Adhesions   —   < 1/3   - 16*
L. OVARY
Deep Endo   —   < 1 cm   -4
Dense Adhesions   —   < 1/3   -4
       TOTAL POINTS   30

PERITONEUM
Superficial Endo   —   > 3cm   - 4
L. OVARY
Deep Endo   —   1-3cm   - 32**
Dense Adhesions   —   < 1/3   - 8**
L. TUBE
Dense Adhesions   —   < 1/3   - 8**
       TOTAL POINTS   52

*Point assignment changed to 16
**Point assignment doubled

PERITONEUM
Deep Endo   —   > 3cm   - 6
CULDESAC
Complete Obliteration   - 40
R. OVARY
Deep Endo   —   1-3cm   - 16
Dense Adhesions   —   < 1/3   - 4
L. TUBE
Dense Adhesions   —   > 2/3   - 16
L. OVARY
Deep Endo   —   1-3cm   - 16
Dense Adhesions   —   > 2/3   - 16
       TOTAL POINTS   114

Determination of the stage or degree of endometrial involvement is based on a weighted point system. Distribution of points has been arbitrarily determined and may require further revision or refinement as knowledge of the disease increases.

To ensure complete evaluation, inspection of the pelvis in a clockwise or counterclockwise fashion is encouraged. Number, size and location of endometrial implants, plaques, endometriomas and/or adhesions are noted. For example, five separate 0.5cm superficial implants on the peritoneum (2.5 cm total) would be assigned 2 points. (The surface of the uterus should be considered peritoneum.) The severity of the endometriosis or adhesions should be assigned the highest score only for peritoneum, ovary, tube or culdesac. For example, a 4cm superficial and a 2cm deep implant of the peritoneum should be given a score of 6 (not 8.) A 4cm deep endometrioma of the ovary associated with more than 3cm of superficial disease should be scored 20 (not 24.).

In those patients with only one adnexa, points applied to disease of the remaining tube and ovary should be multiplied by two. **Points assigned may be circled and totaled. Aggregation of points indicates stage of disease (minimal, mild, moderate, or severe).

The presence of endometriosis of the bowel, urinary tract, fallopian tube, vagina, cervix, skin etc., should be documented under "additional endometriosis." Other pathology such as tubal occlusion, leiomyomata, uterine anomaly, etc., should be documented under "associated pathology." All pathology should be depicted as specifically as possible on the sketch of pelvic organs, and means of observation (laparoscopy or laparotomy) should be noted.

ADJUNCTIVE DIAGNOSTIC PROCEDURES

Ultrasound: Ultrasound is especially valuable for the
evaluation of adnexal masses. Endometriomas usually present as
predominantly cystic masses with variably thickened irregular walls.
Internal echos can give an appearance or a mixed or solid lesion
with or without septae. A differential diagnosis must include
possible ovarian malignancy.

Intravenous Pyelogram (IVP): The evaluation of possible
ureteral involvement should be undertaken in any patient who has
moderate or severe endometriosis. Also, any patients with evidence
of endometriosis overlying a ureter, especially deep in an ovarian
fossa, should be screened with an IVP. Of patients with
endometriosis, 16% have been found to have ureteral involvement.
More importantly, 25% of kidneys with ureteral obstruction from
endometriosis are nonfunctional at the time of diagnosis.

Barium Enema/Colonoscopy: The evaluation of intestinal
involvement by endometriosis should involve barium enema and/or
colonoscopy. This is especially important in patients with a
history of rectal bleeding or severe bowel symptoms.

STAGING

There have been a number of classification systems for
endometriosis. The present system utilized by most gynecologists
was developed by the American Fertility Society (See pages 219-220).

TREATMENT

Therapy in endometriosis is aimed at reducing pain and
decreasing infertility. Treatment must be individualized for each
patient. Factors to be considered include the age of the patient,
the extent of her disease, her desire for fertility or pain relief,
history of previous therapy, contraindications to medical or
surgical therapies, the duration and degree of symptoms, and whether
this represents primary or recurrent endometriosis.

Modern operative laparoscopic techniques have made the
diagnostic laparoscopy a pivotal part of all therapeutic
considerations. Using a multiple puncture technique in combination
with laparscopic instrumentation (unipolar and bipolar cautery
and/or laser vaporization techniques), all minimal and mild
endometriosis as well as a good percentage of moderate endometriosis
can be adequately treated. A comparison of laparoscopic and
laparotomy approaches is presented in the following table:

Conservative Surgery for Endometriosis

	Laparoscopy	Laparotomy
Removal of Peritoneal Implants	Excellent	Good
Lysis of Adhesions	Good	Excellent
Resection of Endometriosis	< 5 cm	$\geq$ 5 cm
Uterine Suspension	Yes	Yes
Neurectomy	Uterosacral Ligament Ablation	Presacral Neurectomy
Intestine, Ureter, Omentum Surgery	No	Yes
Recovery Time	3 - 5 days	4 - 6 weeks

Additional treatment after laparoscopy falls into two categories, medical and surgical.

Medical Therapy: None of the available medical therapies will improve pelvic adhesive disease. Therefore, patients with moderate to severe endometriosis who frequently have significant adhesions will not improve their fertility with medical therapy alone. Contraindications to individual hormonal therapies must be observed.

A. Oral Contraceptives: A progestin dominant pill is recommended to decrease estrogen stimulation to endometrial implants. Oral contraceptives containing Norgestrel work well. Oral contraceptives can be beneficial in the management of dysmenorrhea and dyspareunia in the young patient who does not desire immediate fertility.

B. Progestins: Progestins exert a direct suppressive progestational effect on endometrial implants. Progestins can be used in the management of women who cannot take oral contraceptives and in women after hysterectomy for the management of hot flashes. Medroxyprogesterone acetate, 10-30 mg orally per day or parenteral medroxyprogesterone (Depo-provera) 100-200 mg intramuscularly every 1-2 months is recommended for treatment. Young patients desiring immediate future fertility should not be treated with Depoprovera as prolonged pituitary suppression with anovulation can last for several months after completing

therapy. Reproductive age group women who are sexually
active and not amenorrheic on these medications should use
a barrier form of contraception. Progestin therapy can
cause edema, malaise, and symptoms of depression.

C. Danazol: Danazol is a synthetic androgen derived from 17
α-ethinyl testosterone. Danazol suppresses ovulatory
function probably by preventing the luteinizing hormone
(LH) surge; decreases sex steroid production by directly
inhibiting enzymes responsible for steroidogenesis; and
acts directly on the endometriotic implant by binding the
steroid hormone receptors. Danazol is given in doses of
200-800 mg orally per day for 3-6 months of therapy.
Although various doses have been effective in the treatment
of endometriosis, a state of amenorrhea should be
established and maintained during therapy. Patients on
danazol should use barrier contraception at least until an
amenorrheic state is achieved. Danazol has been used
effectively as a preoperative medication to prepare
patients with severe endometriosis for definitive surgical
therapy. Danazol has not been found to be effective in the
treatment of endometriomas $\geq$ 5 cm in diameter. A number of
androgenic side effects are associated with the use of
danazol therapy including acne, hirsutism, weight gain,
voice changes, and decreased breast size. Occasional other
reactions include gastrointestinal disturbances, weakness,
skin rashes, headaches, and muscle cramps.

D. Gonadotropin-Releasing Hormone Analogues (GnRH analogues):
Analogues of the hypothalamic hormone GnRH have been
formulated to provide a longer biologic half-life. These
long-acting analogues will bind to the pituitary and cause
"down regulation" leading to suppression of LH and follicle
stimulating hormone (FSH) output. Lack of gonadotropin
output will then cause a medical menopause to occur with
severe suppression of endogenous estrogen production.
Although not yet available for general usage, preliminary
studies have shown these analogues to be effective when
used as a daily subcutaneous injection, a monthly
subcutaneous depo-injection, and a daily intranasal
application usually for a 4-6 month period. Side-effects
from the use of the GnRH analogues are not androgenic but
the very low estrogen milieu causes significant hot flashes.
These may be treated with simultaneous administration of a
progestin. The theoretical risk of calcium loss from bones
during the period of low estrogen may also be ameliorated
by simultaneous use of a progestin.

SURGICAL THERAPY

After the initial diagnostic/therapeutic laparoscopy, there are three forms of further surgical intervention for endometriosis:

Conservative Surgery: Laparotomy is necessary for patients who have moderate to severe endometriosis with pelvic adhesions and/or ovarian endometriomas greater than 5 cm. Patients who have failed medical and/or laparoscopic therapy previously, who need a presacral neurectomy, or who need evaluation and possible therapy to other organ systems such as the ureter or intestine require laparotomy. Preoperative danazol therapy, magnification with loopes or microscope, and use of laser vaporization are helpful adjuncts for laparotomy.

Second-look Laparoscopy: The technique of second-look laparoscopy 4-6 weeks after a major laparotomy may be beneficial for fertility. A laparoscopic procedure in this time frame allows separation of adhesions that have minimal amounts of fibrin and are still avascular. Second-look laparoscopy also allows close inspection of areas deep in the pelvis where residual endometriosis may have been overlooked. Second-look laparoscopy is especially beneficial for patients who have undergone extensive ovarian surgery as removal of endometriomas can produce significant adhesions.

Radical Surgery: When fertility is no longer a consideration and symptoms warrant further intervention, a more radical surgical approach including hysterectomy and bilateral salpingo-oophorectomy should be considered. In young patients, consideration should be given to sparing one ovary for endogenous hormone output. The patient must be informed, however, that recurrent symptoms may necessitate a second operation for removal of the ovary. In patients who lose both ovaries, consideration should be given to estrogen replacement therapy (conjugated estrogens 0.625 mg/day) 6-12 months after surgery. Progestin therapy (medroxyprogesterone acetate 10-30 mg/day) is recommended during the interim. In the young patient with severe adhesive disease, consideration should be given to in vitro fertilization before recommending a radical surgical approach.

RESULTS OF THERAPY

Pain Relief: Properly chosen therapeutic regimens, medical or surgical, for the treatment of pain assoicated with endometriosis are reportedly successful in 75-100% of cases. Remember the degree of disease involvement does not correlate with degree of pain. The surgical approach should be considered when large endometriomas or significant pelvic adhesive disease is involved.

Infertility Treatment: Studies evaluating the efficacy of various therapeutic regimens for achievement of pregnancy in patients with documented endometriosis are difficult to compare. Problems associated with these studies include differences in classifications schemes for endometriosis; interobserver variation; differences in dosage and length of therapy for medical intervention; differences in surgical technique during surgical intervention; differences in adjunctive therapy; lack of evaluation of other fertility factors; and a paucity of prospective randomized controlled therapeutic trials. Evaluation of the studies published to date, however, indicate the following:

A. Expectant Management: No treatment of patients with laparoscopically documented minimal or mild endometriosis results in approximately 50% pregnacy rate. Monthly fecundity rates are lower than the general population reflecting a relative reduction in fertility potential. Expected management of moderate or severe endometriosis is not recommended.

B. Medical Therapy: Danazol delays conception attempts for 4-6 months and may not improve pregnancy rates in minimal and mild disease. Pregnancy rates in moderate and severe disease are estimated at 40-50% and 25-30%, respectively. Up to 25% of patients have persistent disease documented laparoscopically on the final day of danazol therapy and recurrence rates may be as high as 40% within 2 years after stopping Danazol.

C. Surgical Therapy: A laparoscopic surgical approach is recommended for minimal to mild endometriosis with pregnancy rates estimated between 55% and 70%. A laparotomy surgical approach is needed for many cases of moderate and severe endometriosis to provide adequate adhesiolysis and treatment of ovarian involvement. Postoperative surgical results indicate pregnancy rates of 45-55% and 30-35% for moderate and severe disease respectively. Several studies have found a combination medical-surgical approach helpful, and this is recommended when signficant endometrial implants cannot be removed during surgery. Recurrent rates after surgical therapy may be up to 40%, however, the time to recurrence may be less than with medical therapy.

SUGGESTED READING

Buttram VC Jr, Reiter RC, Ward S: Treatment of endometriosis with danazol: Report of a 6-year prospective study. Fertil Steril 43:353, 1985.

Goldstein DP, deCholnoky C, Emans SJ, Leventhal JM: Laparoscopy in the diagnosis and management of pelvic pain in adolescents. J Reproduc Med 24:251, 1980.

Kane C, Drouin P: Obstructive uropathy associated with endometriosis. Am J Obstet Gyecol 151:207, 1985.

Olive DL, Haney AF: Endometriosis-Associated Infertility: A critical review of therapeutic approaches. Obstet Gynecol Surv 41:538, 1986.

Pittaway DE, Wentz AC: Endometriosis and corpus luteum function - Is there a relationship? J Reproduc Med 29:712, 1984.

Reyniak JV (ed): Pelvic endometriosis. Seminars in Reproductive Medicine Vol 3, No. 4, 1985.

Schmidt CL: Endometriosis: A reappraisal of pathogenesis and treatment. Fertil Steril 44:157, 1985.

Simpson JL, Elias S, Malinak LR, Buttram VC: Heritable aspects of endometriosis. Am J Obstet Gynecol 137:327, 1980.

Steele RW, Dmowski WP, Marmar DJ: Immunologic aspects of human endometriosis. Am J Reproduc Immunol 6:33, 1984.

Chapter 18

Unexplained Infertility

Anne Colston Wentz, M.D.

INTRODUCTION

If an adequate infertility evaluation has been accomplished, then unexplained infertility should be an unusual finding. Evaluation of the six factors as described in earlier chapters will result in a diagnosis in approximately 95% of couples. Further, the prognosis for unexplained infertility is relatively good, with about 35% of couples achieving pregnancy within a year and a cumulative 60% pregnancy rate in couples diagnosed to have unexplained infertility in the 30 months dating from the diagnostic laparoscopy. However, unexplained infertility is frustrating, and the clinician will be asked to evaluate these couples, usually as a second opinion or last-ditch effort.

INITIAL CONSIDERATIONS

1. Was the initial evaluation complete and thorough, with all six factors investigated?
2. Were results and initial interpretations appropriate?
3. Has iatrogenic infertility resulted from inappropriate therapeutic regimens?
4. Has anything changed or intervened since the evaluation?
5. What additional studies might reasonably be instituted?
6. Have new techologies become available for diagnosis and treatment?

The basic infertility evaluation includes investigation of ovulatory, male, mucus/cervical, endometrial/uterine, tubal and peritoneal factors, and minimally would include keeping a basal temperature chart (BTC) to allow proper timing and interpretation of tests; performing a semen analysis and properly timed post coital test (PCT); obtaining a late luteal phase endometrial biopsy; and doing both a hysterosalpingogram and a double-puncture diagnostic laparoscopy. If any of these tests have not been accomplished appropriately, with appropriate interpretations, then the infertility evaluation should be reinstituted, such that proper priorities can be assigned to the various factors, and no further time wasted.

When the infertility history is reviewed, it is important to ask complete details of previous treatment. Infertility factors may change or worsen over time, and some attempts at therapy may actually decrease the chances for conception. Ovulation induction, particularly with clomiphene citrate, may induce cervical mucus or endometrial abnormalities. Adding estrogens, progesterone or hCG may derange normal folliculogenesis. Inseminations may have been improperly timed. It is useful to attempt to find out why therapy did not work. The discontinuation of all empiric treatment is also important.

The practical approach to evaluation of unexplained infertility includes:

1. a thorough basic infertility evaluation
2. studies repeated as needed

Repeat the semen analysis when:

1. the reference laboratory is unknown
2. there has been a change in the male's history
3. over a year has elapsed from past semen analysis
4. any abnormality is/was found in the male's examination

Repeat the post coital test when:

1. there is any discrepancy between PCT and semen analysis
2. no recent post coital test has been recorded
3. there is any question about the previous evaluation, with either the description or the describer imprecise
4. borderline results are recorded
5. any procedure has been done to the cervix since the last PCT (cryosurgery, cautery)
6. Infection not ruled out.

Repeat the endometrial biopsy when:

1. the previous biopsy was not properly timed
2. previous biopsies showed endometritis, granulomatous disease, or foci of lymphocytes
3. temperature charts appear abnormal
4. menstrual patterns have changed or cycles have altered
5. previous slides uninterpretable or biopsy borderline

Repeat the hysterosalpingogram when:

1. previous films are unavailable
2. films or description are technically inadequate
3. a history of pelvic inflammation has occurred since the last x-ray
4. no recent study
5. any surgical procedure has been done since last evaluation

Repeat the laparoscopy when:

1. previous study possibly inadequate, without a double-puncture or without "blue dye" injection
2. suspicious interval history
3. previous laparoscopy showed "minor" abnormalities
4. no follow-up study following a major surgical procedure (lysis of adhesions, endometrial surgery, use of laser)
5. no recent study
6. abnormalities on examination

FURTHER EXTENSIVE EVALUATION

Further evaluation of the male includes evaluation of both sperm transport and "fertilization." Sperm transport may be abnormal because of infection in either husband or wife, or the presence of antisperm antibodies (AsAb) in either or both members. Although fertilization can only be tested using the mature human oocyte, sperm penetration testing can use either the zona-free hamster egg, or the immature human oocyte. Evaluation of the male for hyperprolactinemia, and/or acrosin content of the human sperm may be accomplished.

FURTHER EVALUATION FOR MALE INFERTILITY

1. Sperm performance testing
   a. cervical mucus cross-match
   b. bovine mucus penetration
   c. zona-free hamster egg penetration
   d. immature human oocyte penetration
   e. motility studies with timed exposure photomicrography, video-micrography or laser Doppler velocimetry
2. Acrosin assay
3. Infection work-up
4. Hyperprolactinemia

Sperm performance testing, a sperm penetration test using the zona-free hamster egg, and perhaps an acrosin assay might be used for further evaluation. Evaluation for antisperm antibodies should be undertaken in men who have undergone vasectomy reversal or varicocelectomy, who have had orchitis, epididymitis, or other infection, or who have had any injury to the testis. Both members may be empirically treated with Vibramycin, 100 mg for 10 days, because of the inadequacy of various methods of culture for ureaplasma and/or Chlamydia. When available, the evaluation might include a two-stage in vitro fertilization (IVF) test, using first the sperm penetration assay of the zona-free hamster egg, and then immature human oocytes to evaluate sperms penetration of the zona pellucida. Hyperprolactinemia must be ruled out in the infertile male, although this would be an unusual finding in the absence of impotence.

Additional areas to be evaluated in the female include the endocrine and ovulatory factors, documentation of the physical act of ovulation, and sperm transport studies.

FURTHER EVALUATION OF THE FEMALE

1. Endocrine factors:
   Measure testosterone, dehydroepiandrosterone sulfate (DS), prolactin; consider thyroid function tests.
   Observe temperature patterns on BTC temperature chart for follicular or luteal phase shortening.
2. Evaluation of ovulation:
   Luteinizing hormone (LH) surge timing correlated with ultrasonography
   Investigate for luteinized unruptured follicle syndrome
3. Evaluation for sperm transport:
   Cervical hostility, endometritis, AsAb, immotile cilia syndrome

The luteinized unruptured follicle syndrome may be investigated by timed ultrasound, LH surge detection, and documentation of failure of the follicle to collapse. Aspiration by culdocentesis of peritoneal fluid and assay of progesterone and estradiol is said to be the definitive means of making the diagnosis. Evaluation for subclinical hyperprolactinemia, hyperandrogenism, infectious diseases, and emotional problems are perhaps indicated. Evaluation for female AsAb should be done if the PCT shows clumping or agglutination of sperm, a shaking phenomenon (+ Kremer test), decreased sperm motility in mucus or immotile sperm. Zona pellucida antibodies have been suggested, but there is not presently available a clinical means of testing for these entities. Cul-de-sac

231

aspiration has been used to demonstrate the presence of sperm in peritoneal fluid.

EMPIRIC THERAPY

1. Ovulation stimulation with clomiphene, human menopausal gonadotropins (hMG), or combinations.
2. Intrauterine insemination.
3. In vitro fertilization (IVF) or Gamete Intrafallopian Transfer (GIFT).
4. Antibiotic therapy.

Although empiricism can be inspired, it is more likely to be misleading. Unrealistic expectations, and considerable expense are encountered. Empiric treatment is almost always inappropriate, it may be damaging to fertility particularly if invasive procedures are inappropriately carried out, and it can be emotionally damaging to the couple. Empiric therapy should be viewed as a desperation move, and not as a therapeutic approach. With IVF statistics showing upward of a 20% ongoing-pregnancy rate at the best programs, and since most of the methods of empiric therapy are not associated with pregnancy rates anywhere near this, it should be realistically discussed with the couple that IVF may in the long run be less expensive, less stressful, and more efficacious than the use of other forms of empiric therapy.

IN VITRO FERTILIZATION

IVF should be undertaken in the couple with unexplained infertility, no more than 18 months from the time of laparoscopy, as the expectation of pregnancy at 18 months is less than 20%. IVF is an appropriate means of determining unrecognized infertility factors in the couple with unexplained infertility. IVF is the "ultimate fertilization test," and replaces the use of the immature human oocyte and the zona-free hamster egg. In couples with unexplained infertility, in whom further more extensive approaches have been unrewarding, an IVF attempt is entirely appropriate. There must be, in the female, poor quality oocytes as there are poor quality sperm in the male. Further, tubal transport problems, due to mechanical tubal factors, which may be important in infertility, can be circumvented by IVF.

232

SUGGESTED READING

Aitken RJ, Warner PE, Reid C: Factors influencing the success of sperm-cervical mucus interaction in patients exhibiting unexplained infertility. J Androl 7:3, 1986.

Barnea ER, Holford TR, McInnes DRA: Long-term prognosis of infertile couples with normal basic investigations: A life-table analysis. Obstet Gynecol 66:24, 1985.

Burslem RW, Osborn JC: Unexplained infertility. Br Med J 292:576, 1986.

Coulam CB, Hill LM, Breckle R: Ultrasonic assessment of subsequent unexplained infertility after ovulation induction. Br J Obstet Gynaecol 90:460, 1983.

Harrison RF, O'Moore RR, O'Moore AM: Stress and fertility: Some modalities of investigation and treatment in couples with unexplained infertility in Dublin. Int J Fertil 31:153, 1986.

Moghissi KS, Wallach EE: Unexplained infertility. Fertil Steril 39:5, 1983.

Musich JR, Behrman SJ: Infertility laparoscopy in perspective: Review of five hundred cases. Am J Obstet Gynecol 143:293, 1982.

Rousseau S, Lord J, Lepage Y, Van Campenhout J: The expectancy of pregnancy for "normal" infertile couples. Fertil Steril 40:768, 1983.

Taylor PJ, Leader A, Pattinson HA: Unexplained infertility: A reappraisal. Int J Fertil 30:53, 1985.

Chapter 19

Recurrent Early Pregnancy Wastage

Anne Colston Wentz, M.D.

DEFINITION

Recurrent early pregnancy wastage is defined as the premature spontaneous termination of at least three consecutive pregnancies with or without preceding successful delivery.

Evaluation, however, should be instituted after two early spontaneous abortions. Women with a live-born child in addition to two or three abortions have a better prognosis than those with abortions alone.

INCIDENCE

The incidence of clinically recognized spontaneous miscarriage in the general population approximates 15-20%. Unrecognized early abortion, occurring after implantation but before the clinical diagnosis of pregnancy, may account for about a 35% rate of embryonic mortality. It is unknown how many embryos are lost after fertilization and before implantation; thus, we have little knowledge of the true incidence of early pregnancy wastage.

The incidence of recurrent miscarriage in the general population is about 0.41%. The likelihood of a second or a third miscarriage remains a controversial statistic, and the risk of a subsequent abortion after three spontaneous losses has been reported to be as high as 47%. However, more optimistic figures have been proposed, which suggest that a patient who has had one abortion should be reassured, but one who has had two consecutive early miscarriages, or a total of three miscarriages interspersed with normal pregnancies, has an increased likelihood of another pregnancy loss, and deserves evaluation. The spontaneous "cure rate" is relatively high, but a search for the etiology is still rewarding.

Empiric Data Concerning the Risks of Spontaneous Abortion
Following a Given Number of Abortions

No. of Previous Abortions	% of Abortions
0	12.3
1	23.7
2	26.2
3	32.2
4	25.9

From data of Warburton and Fraser. Am J Hum Genet 16:1, 1964.

ETIOLOGY OF RECURRENT EARLY PREGNANCY WASTAGE

A. Genetic/Chromosomal
   1. About 50-60% of spontaneous abortions have a chromosomal anomaly.
   2. A balanced translocation will be found in less than 3% of parents with early pregnancy wastage.
   3. The chance of translocation increases to 15-25% where fetal malformations or abnormal stillborn(s) as well as early abortions have been diagnosed.
B. Hormonal
   1. Luteal phase inadequacy: diagnosed in 23-50% of couples depending on author, criteria and population
C. Anatomic, Uterine/Cervical Abnormalities
   1. Uterine anomalies, myomata
   2. Endometrial sclerosis, synechiae
   3. Uterine polyps, other local abnormalities
   4. Incompetent cervix (unusual cause of REPW)
D. Infectious Disease
   1. Acute disease (unlikely cause of REPW)
   2. Chronic disease
      a. Mycoplasma, ureaplasma
      b. Chlamydia
      c. Brucellosis
      d. Listeriosis
E. Metabolic/Endocrine/Chronic Disease
   1. Thyroid, diabetes, adrenal
   2. Renal, hepatic, cardiac
   3. Collagen vascular disease: lupus erythematosis
   4. Sickle cell
F. Immunologic

      1. Antisperm antibodies (AsAb)
      2. HLA compatibility
      3. ABO (?), minor blood group: anti-P
      4. Endometriosis
  G. Iatrogenic
      1. Medications: antimetabolites, other "poisons," alcohol
      2. Progestational agents
      3. Luteolytic agents
  H. Male Factor
      1. Hyperspermia
      2. Oligospermia

Genetic Factor

Distribution of Chromosome Anomalies Among Spontaneous Abortuses

TRISOMY (ALL AUTOSOMES, ESPECIALLY +13, +16, +18, +21)	42.1%
MONOSOMY X (45,X)	23.8%
TRIPLOIDY (3n = 69)	15.5%
TETRAPLOIDY (4n = 92)	4.2%
OTHER	14.4%

Most early spontaneous abortions are caused by chromosomal rearrangements of the conceptus. Recurrent aneuploidy (numerical chromosomal abnormalities) accounts for some repetitive abortions. If the index abortus has a normal karyotype, the second is likely to have a normal karyotype; and similarly, if the initial abortus is abnormal, the second has an 80% chance of being chromosomally abnormal.

In the general population, a balanced translocation, in which there is a mutual exchange of broken-off fragments between chromosomes, occurs with an incidence of about 1.90 per 1000. However, of couples with two or more spontaneous abortions, almost 3% will be found to have balanced reciprocal translocations. If the couples have had both early abortion and fetal malformation, a 27% incidence of cytogenetically abnormal parents is discovered.

Despite the expense, a genetic analysis of both parents is warranted after two abortions. Karyotypic analysis might be attempted on any tissue passed or obtained at curettage after a second early miscarriage and should certainly be performed in a third. Genetic counseling is offered to such couples, and even parents found to have a translocation have a high likelihood of having a normal child.

Hormonal Etiology

About 23-50% of patients with early spontaneous miscarriage have luteal phase inadequacy, defined as endometrial development inadequate to permit or maintain early implantation. A 90% chance of successful pregnancy is expected with appropriate therapy.

Adequacy of corpus luteum function, specifically progesterone output, is needed both for implantation and for maintenance of an early pregnancy, and an inadequate corpus luteum, with a lower-than-normal progesterone production, may be associated with recurrent miscarriage. The incidence of luteal phase inadequacy in the general population is only about 3%, but is much higher in patients presenting with recurrent abortion. Jones and Delfs found LPI responsible for recurrent miscarriage in 34% of patients. Horta et al reported that patients with habitual abortion had lower-than-normal progesterone levels during the luteal phase; when pregnant, progesterone levels were also lower-than-normal, and these patients again subsequently aborted.

The use of the endometrial biopsy as a bioassay of progesterone output has proved satisfactory to make the diagnosis of luteal phase inadequacy (LPI). In one study, 38% of women with three or more consecutive abortions had a poorly developed secretory endometrium compared with an incidence of 6% in infertile women; in another inadequate luteal phase was found in 53% of women with two, and 67% of women with three consecutive miscarriages.

Anatomic Uterine/Cervical Factor

Anatomic uterine defects
double uterus, septate uterus
submucous fibroids, polyps, or uterine synechiae
Incompetent cervical os, either traumatic or congenital

Most mechanical factors cause late abortion, after 12 weeks, although synechiae may interfere with implantation and early placental development. The true rates of pregnancy wastage with anomalous uteri are unknown because many abnormal uteri are never detected and carry normal pregnancies. The rate of pregnancy wastage when a bicornuate uterus has been previously detected is 34%, a septate uterus 22%, and a single uterine horn, 35%; the time of pregnancy wastage is distributed through 3 trimesters, with early abortion being unusual, and premature delivery relatively more common. Each pregnancy with a double uterus is characteristically carried longer than the preceding one.

Submucous fibroids, endometrial polyps, or uterine synechiae which distort the endometrial cavity may also cause repeated abortion.

The incompetent cervical os is characterized by sudden expulsion of a normal sac and fetus between the 18th and 32nd week of pregnancy without prior cramps or bleeding. The factor seems to be more prevalent in those areas of the world where abortion is frequent or obstetrical care, at delivery, poor.

Infectious Disease Factor

Both uterine and disseminated infections have been etiologically related to miscarriage. Among these, viral infections, herpes, rubella, and cytomegalic inclusion disease have been implicated in causing a single miscarriage; listeria, toxoplasmosis, Brucella, Mycoplasma, and perhaps Chlamydia have been implicated in causing recurrent miscarriages.

Metabolic/Endocrine Etiologic Factors

Any chronic disease, toxic environmental exposure, metabolic or endocrine disease can be associated with frequent miscarriage. Hepatic and renal disorders more commonly result in anovulation and not recurrent abortion, but exposure to anesthetic gases and volatile fumes may be associated with both miscarriage or fetal anomalies.

Hypothyroidism is a rare and subtle cause of recurrent miscarriage, but should be suspected clinically and diagnosed by measuring thyroid stimulating hormone (TSH). Only late-stage diabetes mellitus is associated with recurrent miscarriage, and although diabetic patients may have an increased incidence of bacteriuria, the connection with abortion has not been established.

Collagen vascular diseases are associated with recurrent early pregnancy wastage, and systemic lupus erythmatosis (SLE) should always be considered. Recently, a series of circulating antibodies have been described which are involved in the mechanism of abortion; although initially identified in lupus patients, these antibodies have now been found in patients with recurrent fetal wastage who do not have lupus. The lupus anticoagulant, which causes placental thrombosis, is one of these and anticardiolipin (ACL), anti-DNA and other antiphospholipid antibodies have been described.

Immunologic Factors

Immunologic factors are rare causes of recurrent miscarriage. Circulating blocking antibody may protect the fetus against attack by maternal lymphocytes, and patients with habitual abortion may lack appreciable levels of this blocking factor. Human chorionic gonadotropin (hCG) appears to be a suppressant of lymphocytes. If the trophoblast was unable to produce sufficient HCG, possibly because of inadequate progesterone support or inadequate placentation, then possibly a failure of immunologic suppression could result in miscarriage.

Studies of couples with recurrent early pregnancy wastage suggest that these couples share more major histocompatibility complex antigens than do normal child- bearing couples. If couples share HLA antigens, then blocking antibodies may not be generated, and the pregnancy rejected. Data from McIntyre and Faulk, and from Beer, suggest that HLA sharing is significantly more prevalent between couples who suffer from recurrent early fetal wastage. Others have found that fertile couples also share HLA antigens.

Some abortion-prone couples do not share HLA, but mixed lymphocyte culture (MLC) testing of these husband/wife combinations reveals that the wife responds less well to her husband's lymphocytes than to cells from a third party control. Both groups have been treated with leukocyte sensitization therapy. The scientific basis for treating primary chronic aborters with leukocyte transfusions from random donors stems from the discovery that trophoblast/lymphocyte cross-reactive (TLX) antigens are allotypic. Maternal recognition of the allotypic TLX antibodies may be responsible for stimulating a protective or blocking maternal response during normal pregnancy. Couples who share HLA more often may also share TLX, and thus a mother not receiving adequate TLX stimulation would be at high risk for spontaneous recurrent abortion.

Iatrogenic Factors

Iatrogenic causes of recurrent miscarriage include the administration of certain chemotherapeutic and/or cytotoxic agents; colchicine, used in the treatment of gout; and luteolytic agents including progestational agents and estrogens. Alcohol has clearly been shown to be fetotoxic, although drinking must be a rare cause of recurrent early pregnancy wastage.

Male Factors

Both hyperspermia, greater than 250,000,000 sperm/cc, and oligospermia have been associated with frequent miscarriage. This may be secondary to a decreased DNA content of the sperm, but this theory has not been substantiated.

PRECONCEPTIONAL EVALUATION OF COUPLES WITH RECURRENT EARLY FETAL WASTAGE

A. Detailed history, physical and pelvic examination
B. Barrier contraception (diaphragm, condom and foam, sponge) must be used during the evaluation, and until the couple is cleared for pregnancy.
C. Karyotypic analysis of husband and wife
D. Timed endometrial biopsy to assess luteal phase adequacy
E. Hysterosalpingogram
F. Antinuclear antibody (ANA), lupus anticoagulant (LAC), anti cardiolipin (ACL) blood tests to screen for circulating antibodies.
G. Consider obtaining: thyroid function tests; complete blood count (CBC) and serum chemistries; blood group and Coombs; HLA typing, Mycoplasma and Chlamydia culture and/or titers; lupus anticoagulant, or activated partial thromboplastin time, cardiolipin, or activated partial thromboplastin inhibition test.
H. Sperm count.

The history includes a detailed list of prior miscarriages, including actual documentation of the pregnancy, its duration, pathologic description, autopsy reports, and chromosomal studies if performed; note the presence or absence of cramping and bleeding, a description of the labor and the occurrence of any physical or emotional trauma before the occurrence of the abortion; and records preceding illnesses or operations, chronic or acute infection, weight change, drug intake, or illness prior to conception or during early pregnancy. A family history of miscarriages, abortions, congenital anomalies, heritable diseases, consanguinity, stillbirths, and infertility should be mentioned.

The physical examination looks for evidence of acute or chronic illness, endocrinopathy or infection, myomata or the "broad-shouldered" fundus suggestive of a septate uterus. Cervical lacerations, a double vagina, double cervix, or other congenital abnormalities suggestive of mullerian fusion problems should be noted. The passage of a No. 8 Hegar dilator without pain into the endometrial cavity may suggest an incompetent internal cervical os.

The preconceptional evaluation ordinarily will include (1) a karyotypic analysis of both husband and wife, (2) evaluation of luteal phase adequacy by late luteal phase endometrial biopsy, and (3) the performance of a hysterosalpingogram.

The chromosomal analysis should include routine karyotyping, G-banding (Giemsa), C-banding, and fluorescent banding studies. Although numerical aberrations are more common in the population, structural chromosomal abnormalities, including both reciprocal and Robertsonian translocations are an important cause of recurrent miscarriage.

Diagnosis of luteal phase inadequacy is made most easily by taking an endometrial biopsy timed to be obtained within 2-3 days of the expected period. The histologic date must then be correlated with the next menstrual period. If the patient's next menstrual period occurs, for example, the next day after the biopsy was obtained, the histologic pattern of the endometrium should be equivalent to a secretory day 27 pattern, which reflects approximately 13 days of progesterone exposure. If however, the endometrial biopsy is read as earlier, for instance secretory day 21-22, then the biopsy is out-of-phase, reflecting the histologic pattern expected from a shorter duration of progesterone exposure. Thus, the endometrial biopsy is a bioassay of progesterone output. For a valid diagnosis of luteal phase inadequacy, a biopsy out of phase by 2 or more days must be obtained in two or more cycles.

A hysterosalpingogram will diagnose Mullerian anomalies, Asherman's syndrome, polyps or submucous myomata. Mullerian abnormalities occur in one of every 700 women and about 10% of women presenting with habitual abortion will ultimately require a corrective operative procedure. The suggested surgical procedure, if required, for a bicornuate uterus is a Strassman unification, and either the Tompkins or the Jones procedure for a septate uterus. Endometrial sclerosis may be approached by hysteroscopic lysis of adhesions, followed by insertion of either an IUD, or Foley catheter, with estrogenic hormonal support.

The remaining aspects of the preconceptional evaluation include diagnosing and ruling out other less common etiologic factors. A test for ANA and for lupus anticoagulant particularly if the ANA is positive is indicated; recurrent early pregnancy wastage may be the only abnormality in a woman subsequently diagnosed to have lupus. HLA typing and MLC testing may be needed. A CBC, serum chemistries including liver and renal function tests, thyroid studies, and blood group and Coomb's tests on husband and wife may be indicated. TORCH studies including titers for toxoplasmosis, rubella, cytomegalovirus, and herpes are rarely useful. Chronic endometritis should have been diagnosed by the endometrial biopsy used to rule out luteal phase inadequacy. A menstrual collection is needed to diagnose tuberculous endometritis. The cervical mucus or the male

seminal ejaculate may be cultured for <u>Mycoplasma</u>, but both fertile
and pregnant patients may have positive cultures. A semen analysis
for hyper- or oligospermia may be indicated; abnormalities of sperm
morphology may indicate the possibility of environmental toxins.

THERAPEUTIC MODALITIES

    A. Genetic counseling
    B. Progesterone, HCG, rarely clomiphene citrate
    C. Strassman, Tompkins, or Jones unification; other indicated
       operative procedures
    D. Antibiotics

The etiologic cause of recurrent early pregnancy wastage will
be discovered in approximately 70% of presenting couples.

If a genetic etiology is uncovered, the likelihood of having a
live-born child is still relatively high, but obviously depends upon
the chromosomal abnormality diagnosed. Genetic counselling is
required, and a couple can be provided accurate information about
the expectation of a normal or abnormal pregnancy.

If luteal phase inadequacy is diagnosed, treatment with
progesterone supplementation has provided convenient and adequate
correction of the endometrial defect. Progesterone support must be
instituted <u>before</u> the missed menses, as early in the luteal phase as
practical, <u>but care</u> must be taken not to inhibit ovulation.
Beginning treatment on the 3rd day after a temperature rise beyond
97.8°F is usually safe.

Repeat biopsy in the first treated cycle is essential to ensure
correction of the defect. About 13% of treated patients do not have
an adequate endometrial pattern with the approach to treatment.

POST CONCEPTIONAL AND EARLY PREGNANCY MANAGEMENT

    A. Useful procedures
       1. Early diagnosis
       2. Accurate dates
          BTC
       3. Serial quantitative β-hCG
          doubling time
       4. Ultrasonography
       5. Plan to karyotype products of conception
          at D & C for incomplete abortion;
          if no development diagnosed by ultrasonography
            and β-hCG

242

- B. Uncertain usefulness
    1. Serial TSH, T_4, T_3
    2. Avoidance of stress
    3. Avoidance of intercourse
    4. Serial serum progesterone levels
    5. Culture of products of conception
        ureaplasma, <u>Mycoplasma</u>
- C. Myths
    1. Bedrest

A barrier method of contraception is necessary during evaluation, and until the cycle is cleared for pregnancy. The proper therapy is instituted, perhaps genetic counselling or a surgical approach. If LPI was diagnosed, then correction of the defect with progesterone supplementation is documented before pregnancy is attempted. The BTC should be continued, such that a pregnancy may be diagnosed as early as possible. The patient should be instructed to report delayed menses immediately.

The quantitative measurement of β-hCG is helpful, and 3 hCG measurements taken at 2-day intervals is used to calculate the hCG doubling time which may indicate normal or abnormal hCG output. The normal doubling time of β-hCG in early pregnancy varies between 1.6 and 2.5 days. A pregnancy with low hCG titers should not be supported with progesterone to avoid masking a missed abortion or intrauterine fetal death. A normal doubling time does not guarantee normality.

Progesterone in very early pregnancy decreases from the time of the missed period until approximately 6-7 weeks from the last menstrual period; even serial values may be shown to be normally decreasing at this stage of gestation. However, if values are below 10 ng/ml, virtually no patient will maintain the pregnancy. Sequential ultrasonography, and frequent examinations to determine both gestational size and cervical dilatation, may be in order.

The determination of TSH, T_4, T_3, and T_3 uptake may be indicated, as subclinical hypothyroidism may be responsible for early miscarriage. Coitus during early pregnancy may be inadvisable as the male seminal ejaculate contains prostaglandins in concentrations which can cause uterine contractions in both the nonpregnant and pregnant uterus. Additionally, orgasm is ordinarily associated with increased uterine motility and measurable uterine contractions.

Even if an etiologic cause has been determined and appropriately treated, for instance a double uterus unified, or a luteal phase defect supported by progesterone administration, subsequent miscarriage may occur due to a sporadic genetic cause. If 50-60% of all spontaneous miscarriages are caused by random genetic abnormalities, then a single miscarriage may have this etiology. The attempt should be made to karyotype the fetal tissue from the subsequent miscarriage.

Vaginal bleeding especially if accompanied by cramping is always of concern. Up to 50% of pregnant women will bleed early in pregnancy, and of those with significant bleeding, about 60-70% will ultimately abort. Bed rest is useful psychologically. Importantly, progesterone or a progestational agent administered at this time will not prevent the occurrence of miscarriage. A recent study of threatened abortion randomized progestational agent treatment in patients diagnosed and followed by ultrasound. The finding was that approximately 70% of patients with a threatened abortion ultimately aborted, and there was no difference between treated and untreated groups. However, treating with the progestational drug significantly prolonged the time before abortion occurred.

Good obstetrical management includes correction of nutritional deficiencies, administration of vitamin and iron supplementation, avoidance of communicable infections in the prospective mother, and emotional support.

Finally, recurrent early fetal wastage may result from emotional factors, and abruptio placenta is commonly seen in patients under emotional or psychological stress. If no other factors explaining recurrent abortion can be identified, counseling, and the awareness of the importance of emotional factors, may change the outcome in a particular case.

To conclude, prognosis in recurrent early pregnancy wastage is excellent, if a diagnosis has been achieved and therapy properly directed.

SUGGESTED READING

Andrews T, Dunlop W, Roberts DF: Cytogenetic studies in spontaneous abortuses. Hum Genet 66:77, 1984.

Beer AE, Quebbeman JF, Ayers JWT, Haines RF: Major histocompatibility complex antigens, maternal and paternal immune responses, and chronic habitual abortions in humans. Am J Obstet Gynecol 141:987, 1981.

244

Caudle MR, Rote NS, Scott JR, DeWitt C, Barney MF: Histocompatibility in couples with recurrent spontaneous abortion and normal fertility. Fertil Steril 39:793, 1983.

Fine LG, Barnett EV, Danovitch GM, Nissenson AR, Conolly ME, Lieb SM, Barrett CT: Systemic lupus erythematosus in pregnancy. Ann Intern Med 94:667, 1981.

FitzSimmons J, Jackson D, Wapner R, Jackson L: Subsequent reproductive outcome in couples with repeated pregnancy loss. Am J Med Genet 16:583, 1983.

Fizet D, Bousquet J: Absence of a factor blocking a cellular cytotoxicity reaction in the serum of women with recurrent abortions. Brit J Obstet Gynaecol 90:453, 1983.

Glass RH, Golbus MS: Habitual abortion. Fertil Steril 29:257, 1978.

Hensleigh PA, Fainstat T: Corpus luteum dysfunction: serum progesterone levels in diagnosis and assessment of therapy for recurrent and threatened abortion. Fertil Steril 32:396, 1979.

McIntyre JA, McConnachie PR, Taylor CG, Faulk WP: Clinical, immunologic, and genetic definitions of primary and secondary recurrent spontaneous abortions. Fertil Steril 42:849, 1984.

Neri G, Serra A, Campana M, Tedeschi B: Reproductive risks for translocation carriers: cytogenetic study and analysis of pregnancy outcome in 58 families. Am J Med Genet 16:535, 1983.

Simpson JL: Genes, chromosomes, and reproductive failure. Fertil Steril 33:107, 1980.

Taylor C, Faulk WP: Prevention of recurrent abortion with leucocyte transfusions. Lancet 1:68, 1981.

Thi Tho P, Byrd JR, McDonough PG: Etiologies and subsequent reproductive performance of 100 couples with recurrent abortion. Fertil Steril 32:398, 1979.

Chapter 20

Basics of *in Vitro* Fertilization (IVF), Gamete Intrafallopian Transfer (GIFT), Other New Technologies

Anne Colston Wentz, M.D.

BASICS OF IN VITRO FERTILIZATION

Human in vitro fertilization (IVF) has become a widely accepted method of treatment for infertile couples. The original studies were carried out primarily in England by Drs. Robert Edwards and Patrick Steptoe, culminating in the first live human birth in their program in 1978. In the United States, the first baby born from an IVF attempt was delivered on December 28, 1981, from the efforts of Drs. Howard and Georgeanna Jones of the Eastern Virginia Medical School in Norfolk. Over the past several years, there has been a marked increase in the number of programs established in the United States and around the world, and by early 1987, over 3000 live births have been recorded.

INDICATIONS FOR IN VITRO FERTILIZATION

1. Fallopian Tube Obstruction
2. Oligospermia
3. Abnormal cervical factor
4. Immunologic factor - husband or wife
5. Unexplained infertility
6. Persistent infertility after tubal surgery
7. Persistent infertility after treatment for endometriosis

Initially, IVF was designed for patients with severe tubal disease. However, with pregnancy rates about 20% per transfer, the technique has been expanded as treatment for other problems. Male factor infertility, oligospermia, is an area of particular interest, as fertilization in vitro can be accomplished with fewer sperm than apparently necessary in vivo.

CRITERIA FOR INCLUSION

1. Clear-cut indication for IVF
2. Records available to the IVF team
3. Ability to communicate (foreign language, translation)
4. Ability to understand the IVF procedure, cryopreservation, and other modifications
5. Capable of informed consent

STAGES OF IVF

1. Pretreatment screening of couple
2. Patient selection
3. Choice of stimulation protocol
4. Induction of timed superovulation
5. Monitoring of follicular development
6. Ovum recovery
7. Laboratory techniques and IVF
8. Growth of embryo in culture
9. Embryo placement or transfer
10. Luteal phase monitoring
11. Diagnosis of pregnancy
12. Analyzing reasons for failure
13. Obstetrical care
14. Psychological considerations

1. Pretreatment screening of couple: considerations
   A. Areas to be evaluated, screened or discussed
      1) surgical
         a. percentage of ovarian access
         b. one versus two ovaries
         c. decision of route of oocyte aspiration (laparoscopy, percutaneous transvesicle ultrasound-guided [USG] aspiration, transvaginal USG aspiration)
         d. need for mini-lap
      2) medical
         a. contraindications to outpatient laparoscopy or USG aspiration
            Anesthesia clarification
            Weight: less than 150% ideal body weight
         b. Rubella immunity
      3) psychological
         a. ability to withstand stress
         b. appropriate motivation
      4) social
         a. employment assured
         b. pressures at home or work identified and dealt with

                5) financial
                    a. ability to afford the procedure
                    b. insurance coverage optimized
        B. Screening laparoscopy
                1) usually not needed
        C. Additional information:
                1) uterine position and normality
                2) uterine depth and direction
                3) characteristics of endocervical canal
                4) menstrual cycle regularity

        Much of the pretreatment screening of the couple comes from
medical records, and from telephone interview, if the couple is
coming from a distance for IVF. A discussion of the risks and
benefits of laparoscopy in an unknown pelvis is essential. The
couple needs to know the team's favored oocyte aspirate technique,
whether laparoscopic or USG, and in the latter situation, whether
the transabdominal or transvaginal route is used. The medical record
and the patient interview attempt to establish whether the patient
is appropriate for an outpatient anesthetic and has no medical
contraindications to the operative procedure. The degree of pelvic
adhesion formation, and whether the patient has one or two ovaries
may determine what stimulation protocol is used, for IVF teams use
different stimulations for different situations. Ovarian
accessibility may affect whether laparoscopic aspiration is tried,
or whether a percutaneous transvesicle USG needle aspiration is
attempted. Also part of the pretreatment screening of the couple is
a psychological and social evaluation, as patients do not realize
until they are told about the financial and emotional stresses of
IVF.

        The evaluation of the male is also part of the initial
screening, as a semen analysis (SA) performed by a competent
laboratory is important. Whether or not a sperm penetration assay
(human sperm penetration of a zona-free hamster egg as a test of
"fertilizing capacity") is required is individually determined.

        Additional information about the wife includes confirmation of
a presumptively ovulatory menstrual cycle, rubella immunity, some
information about the normality of the uterine cavity, and perhaps a
pretreatment screening laparoscopy performed either by the IVF team
or a physician known to provide detailed information about pelvic
adhesion formation and ovarian access.

2. Patient Selection

        Patients to be considered for IVF should have undergone a
complete infertility investigation with correction where possible of

abnormalities. Such an approach will not only achieve pregnancy
without the need for IVF in significant numbers of patients, but
also identify the specific abnormalities which will make the patient
either a good or a poor candidate for IVF.

The major categories of abnormality considered for the
procedure include irreparable tubal damage, unexplained infertility,
a relative male factor, and endometriosis. Several other categories
of patients currently being evaluated for the efficacy of IVF
include immunologic factors, cervical factors, and those with
ovulatory dysfunction who fail to conceive with appropriate
treatment. The success of IVF in these patients remains unknown.
Preliminary data suggest that the prognosis for success is best in
patients with tubal damage as the only barrier to fertility.
Patients with endometriosis may also do well, but the number of
patients reported in this category is small. Couples with
unexplained infertility and male factor seem to be less successful.

In addition to a careful review of the previous infertility
evaluation, in depth patient counseling as to the cost, effort,
stress, and realistic success prognosis should be carried out with
all patients. If a serious emotional instability is present,
psychiatric consultation is indicated prior to acceptance into the
program; however, most patients entering IVF programs are remarkably
emotionally healthy and stable, considering their past histories.

3. Choice of Stimulation Protocol

    A.   None - Normal cycle + human chorionic gonadotropin (hCG)
    B.   Clomiphene citrate (CC) + hCG
    C.   Human menopausal gonadotropins + hCG
    D.   Clomiphene + hMG + hCG
    E.   Pure follicle stimulating hormone (FSH) + hCG
                                              + hMG + hCG
                                              + CC + hCG
                                              + hMG + CC + hCG
    F.   Pulsatile GnRH + hCG

4. Induction of Timed Superovulation

There are three basic protocols for follicular stimulation of
ovulatory patients. The intent is to induce development of a
maximum number of follicles containing mature oocytes to be
aspirated prior to ovulation.

CC. CC, 50-150 mg daily for 5 days is given beginning on days
2-5 of the cycle. Monitoring of estradiol (E_2) levels and

follicular development by ultrasound is begun about the 7th day from beginning the drug. HCG is given when follicular diameter measures 17 mm or more, two or more follicles are seen and E_2 levels have peaked. Laparoscopy is planned for 35 hours following the hCG injection. Ultrasound is usually performed the morning of surgery, and laparoscopy is cancelled if the ultrasound shows that ovulation has already occurred.

HMG. Two or more ampules of hMG are administered beginning cycle days 2-5 with daily E_2 and ultrasound examinations beginning around cycle day 6. Flexible or fixed treatment regimens are used, and some teams use a divided hMG administration, with 1-2 ampules injected twice daily. Pulsatile hMG administration is also being evaluated. HCG is ordinarily stopped when the follicle diameter is 14-15 mm and the E_2 is greater than 600 pg/ml. HCG 2500-10000 IU is given 24-48 hours later. Laparoscopy follows the hCG injection by approximately 35 hours with a preoperative ultrasound to assure that ovulation has not occurred. Some teams monitor for a premature LH surge using urinary or serum parameters.

CC-hMG. CC is begun as described and hMG is started either concurrently or sequentially. HMG is continued until certain parameters of E_2 and follicular diameter are met. There is considerable variation in protocols used by different teams. The hCG trigger is usually given, although these patients will ovulate spontaneously, and some teams prefer to monitor for the luteinizing hormone (LH) surge and schedule aspiration accordingly.

GnRH Pump. The ability to stimulate multiple follicles with pharmacologic doses of GnRH by pump infusion has been described. This method of ovarian stimulation may come into clinical usefulness in the future, but is unlikely to yield as many oocytes. Improved oocyte maturity but fewer numbers may result, which may be advantageous for those teams not using cryopreservation and which do not want or need excess eggs or embryos.

Pure FSH. "Pure" FSH, without LH content, is being investigated as a superior agent for follicular recruitment and stimulation. Used similar to hMG, pure FSH seems to result in the recruitment and stimulation of more follicles, the capability to aspirate more oocytes, to transfer more embryos and to cause more pregnancies. Multiple gestation may be a problem. For teams not using cryopreservation, excess embryos may not be an advantage.

5. Monitoring of Follicular Development

Although most IVF teams use some combination of follicular detection by ultrasound, measurement of E_2 and LH levels, and occasionally observation of cervical mucus, there is absolutely no consensus as to what constitutes a "good" stimulation and how best to monitor it. This aspect of IVF is the most varied among teams, and each variation has its advocates.

There is better agreement on what constitutes a "poor" stimulation. A low or slow E_2 rise, stimulation of too few and particularly only a dominant follicle, a drop in E_2 before or after the hCG injection, premature LH surge and any adverse reaction to the medication (fever, rash) are indication to terminate the attempt.

6. Ovum Recovery

Various techniques have been used for oocyte aspiration, most of which have used a laparoscopic approach, with at least 2 and more frequently 3 punctures. The aspiration needle may be passed through the operating channel of the laparoscope, or may be used through a separate puncture. Different types of traps and oocyte collection devices are used by various teams. Some use a 50 ml syringe for suction, whereas others use wall suction with 150 mm Hg pressure.

The use of a USG, percutaneous, transvesicle aspiration approach is being used by many groups. Somewhat fewer oocytes may be aspirated, but fertilization and pregnancy rates are quite good. The efficiency of the procedure will probably improve with experience, and will supplant the laparoscopic technique for oocyte pickup. Laparoscopy is considered obsolete by some teams.

Receiving even more enthusiastic favor from physician and patient both is the transvaginal USG approach; intraperitoneal CO_2 is not needed and bladder distention unnecessary. The needle passes through a guide although some use a hand-held approach; the aspiration needle can be spring-loaded for puncture. Oocyte recovery is easily accomplished, and efficiency is apparently quite good.

7. Laboratory techniques and IVF

If the follicle is mature, a visible amount of granulosa cells will accompany the aspirated fluid, in which will be found a mature ovum. The follicular fluid is examined as rapidly as possible under the microscope in the laboratory. The oocyte with its surrounding cumulus is quickly identified, graded as to maturity, and placed in the incubation medium in a dish placed in the incubator. Immature eggs have a tight corona and a small cumulus mass which is not expanded. Mature eggs have a loose corona and an expanded cumulus mass. Several different media are used by different programs, but whatever the medium chosen for follicular aspiration and ovum culture, it should be quality controlled by monitoring the physical parameters of the solution (pH, osmolarity, temperature) as well as the biologic effects on normal mouse embryo development and sperm motility.

The insemination and incubation media used include Ham's F-10, Earle's T-6, and other media, supplemented by heat-inactivated human serum or fetal cord serum or another source of protein. The optimum time in culture prior to insemination for a healthy mature preovulatory oocyte is about 4-8 hours, and for an immature oocyte considerably larger, up to 24 hours usually, and even longer if the polar body has not been expelled.

Various types of sperm preparation are used, from a simple washing and centrifugation, to more complicated "swim-up" procedure which separate only motile sperm to be used for insemination. Insemination is carried out with between 50,000 and 500,000 motile sperm per ml. Various concentrations and total sperm amounts are used by different teams, and it appears that about 50,000/ml is suitable.

8. Growth of embryo in culture

The oocyte is examined some 15-18 hours after insemination, and at this time switched from the incubation to growth medium, which ordinarily contains about double the amount of protein as in the first insemination media. The oocyte is examined for fertilization, suggested but not proven by the appearance of two pronuclei, and two polar bodies. The fertilized oocyte is then returned to the incubator until the time for transfer, which is variable, but usually about 40 hours from insemination. At this time, the fertilized oocyte or zygote or conceptus is ordinarily in the four-cell stage.

Fertilization rates depend on the maturity and normality of the oocyte aspirated. Of healthy, preovulatory mature oocytes, fertilization rates of about 85% are achieved. For immature oocytes, fertilization rates can be expected to be about 50%, but once fertilization has been achieved, cleavage rates are usually greater than 90%.

9. Embryo Placement or Transfer

    A. Timing: 40-70 hours from insemination; 4- to 8-cell stage
    B. Location: close to the laboratory
    C. Patient position: knee-chest or lithotomy

D. Equipment and technique:
    small Teflon catheter
    Tom Cat catheter, 3.5 Fr.
    with or without tenaculum on cervical lip
E. Adjuvant therapy
    antibiotics
    Valium, 10 mg 1 hour before transfer

At approximately 40 hours from insemination, when the embryos have reached the 4- to 6-cell stage, embryo placement is carried out. This is done using different transfer catheters and with different patient positioning. Although the lithotomy position is used by most teams, some teams prefer to place the patient in knee-chest position if her uterus is anterior, and transfer in lithotomy position only for posterior retroflexed uteri.

A small Teflon catheter is usually used, and some teams use a metal cannula to guide the catheter. Gloves are not used in this procedure since powder of all kinds is toxic to embryos. Similarly, all instrumentation is washed only with water and the cervix cleaned with sterile saline. No detergent should be used on any of the apparatus for embryo culture, transfer, or ovum retrieval.

The growth media containing the embryo is expelled into the uterine fundus. Very small amounts of transfer medium are used, 10-70 μl, and there is some debate as to the appropriate volume of transfer medium. Ectopic pregnancies have been reported, but there is also the fear of not expelling the conceptus from the transfer catheter.

10. Luteal Phase Monitoring

Most teams administer progesterone, in injectable or suppository form, during the luteal phase. There is no real support for this practice, as several studies have shown normal progesterone output following aspiration. Nevertheless, intramuscular injection of 12.5-25 mg progesterone is almost universal.

Shorter luteal phase duration has been reported with many of the hyperstimulation protocols. Total luteal phase length from transfer has been reported to be 8-10 days in patients who do not become pregnant.

11. Diagnosis of Pregnancy

A β-hCG will be positive approximately 11 days from transfer if pregnancy has resulted. Transient elevations of hCG have been recorded, which suggests that some implantations begin but do not continue.

Pregnancy rates vary with the IVF team but most report that 20% of transfers result in pregnancy. However, the pregnancy rate is dependent more on the number of oocytes aspirated and the number of embryos transferred than on any other particular factor. In most programs, if one embryo is transferred, a 10% chance of pregnancy results, which increases to about 35% when three or more embryos are transferred.

Pregnancy rates for IVF are now beginning to be as good if not better than, for example, pregnancy rates in the treatment of severe male infertility, or rates following a second operative procedure for correction of tubal infertility. Results can be anticipated to improve, but it appears that larger centers with a higher volume of patients will, over time, have the best results.

12. Analyzing Reasons for Failure

    A. The patient may ovulate prematurely or retrieved ova may fail to fertilize.
    B. Scarring or adhesions may make it impossible to remove an ovum from the ovary. Clearly, all oocytes are not comparable in quality and morphologic criteria are not infallible in determining maturity. Insemination may not have been done at the proper time.
    C. The hormonal milieu may be unfavorable to the oocyte.
    D. The stimulation parameters may not have been as good as possible.
    E. Transferred embryo may fail to implant. This represents the single greatest source of failure at the present time. The factors necessary for implantation to occur and the syncrony between embryo development and endometrium are largely unknown.
    F. The sperm may have been of inadequate quality. The rise motility may have been poor and/or too few sperm recovered from the rise for adequate insemination. The ejaculate may have been infected or contain antisperm antibodies.
    G. Endometrial development may have been deranged or somehow inappropriate for implantation.
    H. The rate of spontaneous abortion seems to be higher for IVF fetuses than for those conceived naturally, and many more chemical pregnancies occur than viable clinical pregnancies.

13. Obstetrical Care

Once a normal pregnancy has been established, obstetrical care is no different than that for any other patient and is based on obstetrical indications. There is no specific IVF-oriented indication for amniocentesis. This is also true for the management of labor and delivery.

14. Psychological Considerations

A critical part of any IVF program is post-treatment counseling and support. Since 80-85 couples out of 100 will fail to conceive on a given cycle, a formal counseling and support process must be carried out to help the couple deal with the grief and frustration of failure. The grief reaction is similar to that for any individual who has lost a pregnancy, as these patients consider themselves pregnant once embryo transfer has occurred. Helping the couple work through these grief reactions is an integral part of the long term healing of the patient regardless of the success or failure of the procedure.

Repeat attempts at IVF for a given couple are limited primarily by the emotional and economic tolerance of the couple. This must be individualized from couple to couple but most will try 3-4 times.

NEW APPROACHES IN REPRODUCTIVE TECHNOLOGY

1. Cryopreservation
2. Embryo Flushing and Transfer
3. The GIFT procedure
4. Donor Eggs

1. Cryopreservation

In most programs, the optimum number of embryos transferred, resulting in the optimum chance for pregnancy, appears to be 3 or 4 healthy 2- to 4-cell conceptuses. If fewer are transferred, the pregnancy rate is less; if more are transferred, there appears to be some inhibitory factor that results in a decreased likelihood of pregnancy. Rarely, there has been the complication of a multiple gestation.

Cryopreservation has theoretical advantages, including the possibility of a decreased cumulative number of cycles to pregnancy, increased cost efficacy, decreased risk of multiple pregnancy, and potential replacement in a natural cycle. As one of the explanations for failure to achieve pregnancy is that hyperstimulation is used in the stimulation cycle, then replacement in a natural cycle has the advantage of no anesthesia, and no adversely increased estradiol and progesterone levels. Finally, there is also the possibility of better assessment of embryo viability, as another reason for failure of implantation could be the possibility of implantation could be the possibility of inadequately healthy eggs and embryos. The viability of blastomeres can be ascertained after thaw before placement of an embryo.

Cryopreservation is done automatically, using one of reversal available programmed freezing units, with or without automatic "seeding" which allows ice crystals to form in a controlled fashion. Slow and fast freezing and thawing regimens are used, and there is on-going work to identify the best cryoprotectant. Embryo viability is graded on the basis of the number of surviving blastomeres; 50% or more are needed for transfer.

2. Embryo Flushing and Transfer

Embryo flushing and transfer has been developed as an alternative to IVF, particularly to be used by those women in whom there is no ovarian access, no ovaries, no chance of oocyte aspiration, and perhaps those with ovarian failure or Turner's syndrome. In this technique, a normally ovulating woman who has been paid to donate her egg is inseminated with the sperm of the husband. Two to five days later, uterine flushing is carried out with a sterile solution, and the cleaved embryo identified in the uterine washings. This embryo is then transferred into the uterus of the recipient, whose husband donated the sperm, but who was unable to contribute an egg. Hormonal preparation would have to be used for women without ovaries, with ovarian failure or Turner's syndrome, but otherwise the embryo would be placed in a normal cycle, approximately 5 days after the LH surge has been identified. As of this writing, there has been limited experience with the technique; two live births have occurred in recipient women, and in women donating the egg, pregnancy necessitating termination has been documented.

3. The GIFT procedure

Gamete intrafallopian tube transfer (GIFT) was developed by Dr. Ricardo Asch in San Antonio, Texas, as an alternative to IVF for women with open fallopian tubes. In this technique, the follicular stimulation, laparoscopy and ovum aspiration or oocyte aspiration is accomplished in an identical manner to IVF. Recently, the GIFT procedure has been facilitated by the use of the minilaparotomy which has the advantage of not requiring a CO_2 pneumoperitoneum, instead of laparoscopy, but the precise technique of aspiration has not been finalized. Without terminating the laparoscopy, a husband's specimen which has undergone washing and/or rise is placed with no more than 4 oocytes, regardless of the number aspirated, and then the resulting insemination medium is divided between the two tubes; the oocyte-sperm combination is placed into the fimbriated end of the tube using a catheter somewhat like a transfer catheter for embryo placement. The laparoscopy is then terminated. Pregnancy rates of 40% have been reported.

The procedure usually generates excess oocytes. These may be inseminated and the embryos cryopreserved, the excess oocytes donated, or the oocytes terminated.

The advantage of the procedure is that it avoids time and culture in the laboratory for oocytes and for sperm. It does however require most of the other techniques of IVF, and the cost will not be greatly decreased.

GIFT without laparoscopy has been accomplished. USG transvaginal oocyte aspiration is done, the eggs and sperm combined, and then introduced through the cervix and uterus and into the fallopian tubal ostium using a specially prepared small catheter. (General anesthesia is not required.)

4. Donor eggs

Donor eggs may be obtained from a number of sources, including women undergoing laparoscopic sterilization, those undergoing IVF from whom an abundance of oocytes have been obtained, and even from women undergoing operative procedures. Eggs can be frozen, or can be immediately donated at the time of the procedure, and inseminated with the husband's sperm. Women requiring donor eggs would be limited to those without ovaries, with Turner's syndrome or ovarian failure, and those in whom ovaries are entirely inaccessible even by ultrasound aspiration techniques.

SUGGESTED READING

Blandau RJ: In vitro fertilization and embryo transfer. Fertil Steril 33:3, 1980.

Johnston I, Lopata A, Speirs A et al: In vitro fertilization: The challenge of the eighties. Fertil Steril 36:699, 1981.

Jones HW: The ethics of in vitro fertilization - 1982. Fertil Steril 37:146, 1982.

Jones HW, Acosta A, Andrews MC, Garcia JE, Jones GS, Mantzavinos T, McDowell J, Sandow B, Veeck L, Whibley T, Wilkes C, Wright G: The importance of the follicular phase to success and failure in in vitro fertilization. Fertil Steril 40:317, 1983.

Jones HW, Acosta A, Garcia JE, Sandow BA, Veeck L: On the transfer of conceptuses from oocytes fertilized in vitro. Fertil Steril 39:241, 1983.

Jones HW, Jones GS, Andrews MC, Acosta A, Bundren C, Garcia J, Sandow B, Veeck L, Wilkes C, Witmyer J, Wortham JE, Wright G: The program of in vitro fertilization at Norfolk. Fertil Steril 38:14, 1982.

Veeck LL, Wortham JWE, Witmyer J, Sandow BA, Acosta AA, Garcia JE, Jones GS, Jones HW: Maturation and fertilization of morphologically immature human oocytes in a program of in vitro fertilization. Fertil Steril 39:594, 1983.

Wortham JWE, Veeck LL, Witmyer J, Sandow BA, Jones HW: Vital initiation of pregnancy (VIP) using human menopausal gonadotropin and human chorionic gonadotropin ovulation induction: Phase II-1981. Fertil Steril 40:170, 1983.

Chapter 21

Psychologic Aspects of Infertility

Anne Colston Wentz, M.D.

The emotional impact of both involuntary infertility as well as its evaluation have been accepted but largely ignored. Infertility profoundly affects the behavioral and emotional relationship of any couple, and there is some suggestion that the stress of these emotional factors might contribute to the infertility.

Cycle of Psychologic Aspects of Infertility

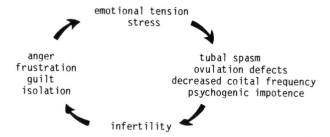

emotional tension
stress

anger
frustration
guilt
isolation

tubal spasm
ovulation defects
decreased coital frequency
psychogenic impotence

infertility

The infertility work-up constitutes a major invasion of privacy. Couples come to the evaluation with varying degrees of anxiety, guilt, a sense of failure, and self-doubt. Infertility erodes a couple's self-esteem and the evaluation further intensifies feelings and focuses attention on those areas which are most painful. Sexual performance and function come under close scrutiny and supervision, with resultant unconscious failure to perform, manifested by broken appointments or psychogenic impotence. Infertile people feel incomplete, defective and abnormal, and the harder they try to change their circumstances, the more frustrated they become. Their world is a constant swing of emotion, from hope, excitement, and anticipation to the despair brought monthly by the onset of menses.

Certain effects of infertility can be clearly recognized. For example, while the sexual functioning of a couple affects their fertility, their infertility also influences their sexual function. Coital frequency may be decreased, or concentrated in midcycle, to the extent that the act becomes work and a necessary performance. The intimacy of sexual intercourse is lost; previously private aspects of marital life are openly discussed, tested, and graded. Sexual dysfunction commonly occurs, and with appropriate questioning, may be found in about 20% of infertile couples. For example, iatrogenic impotence may result from frequent postcoital testing (PCT) and regimented sex. Marital problems can result in extramarital relations to escape the continued feelings of failure. Communication between couples may disappear as the pressure upon one or the other mounts.

Menning views infertility as a life crisis, a disruption in the steady state and a period of disequilibrium. Resolution is the goal of any crisis, and infertile couples facing similar problems express a similar syndrome of feelings.

The "crisis of infertility" requires resolution. The order of feelings to be dealt with are similar to those encountered with the death of a loved one, and are experienced by couples in virtually the same order although with dissimilar intensity. These are:

1. surprise
2. denial
3. anger
4. isolation
5. guilt
6. grief
7. acceptance and resolution

Surprise is not unanticipated for a couple who has become used to thinking in terms of birth control and contraception. Denial follows, particularly for achievement-oriented people who are accustomed to success. Denial is useful because it can provide a time for delaying and slowing down and only becomes a problem itself if it becomes a permanent coping mechanism.

Anger is perhaps the most obvious emotion seen by the infertility specialist. Anger may be rational and reasonable, directed toward indignities of the testing or to the "unfairness" of infertility. More frequently, it is projected onto the physician, the spouse or pregnant friends, and is irrational and unreasonable. This anger needs ventilation, although it frequently replaces other inexpressible feelings such as helplessness, loss of control, or grief.

Isolation is another stage along the line to acceptance, a time when couples are past their anger but unable to come to grips with their infertility. They feel the need for secrecy to avoid painful encounters and withdraw from social contacts. Guilt may be a reason also for the need for secrecy and to withdraw. The couple reviews their lives and experiences searching for the reason for their punishment.

When a couple is able to grieve for their lost fertility, they have begun to accept their situation. Resolution with acceptance is the goal of intervention in the crisis of infertility. This allows the couple to continue their lives, with priorities intact and a perspective of where they have been and where they are going.

Not all infertile couples are able to work through these intense feelings and arrive at resolution. However, the infertility specialist must recognize their existence and be willing to help patients deal with the varied emotions that constitute the crisis of infertility.

What the physician can do to help has also been discussed by Menning:

1. Treat infertility as a problem of the couple.
2. Develop the plan of investigation and treatment with the couple.
3. Offer emotional support and education.
4. Respect the level of one's expertise.
5. Be accessible.
6. Be aware of the existence of support groups-particularly RESOLVE.

SUGGESTED READING

Mahlstedt PP: The psychological component of infertility. Fertil Steril 43:335, 1985.

Menning BE: The emotional needs of infertile couples. Fertil Steril 34:313, 1980.

Sloan D: Psychogenic aspects of infertility. Infertility 5:319, 1982.

Chapter 22

Contraception

Liliana Kossoy, M.D.

FOR THE MALE

CONDOMS

Condoms provide a simple, effective, and reversible method of male contraception with no side-effects. They are inexpensive, easy to obtain and provide protection against sexually transmitted diseases (syphilis, gonorrhea, herpes, Chlamydia) when used in all types of contacts including nongenital to genital as well as throughout coitus. Condom use during pregnancy may protect against amniotic fluid infection.

Effectiveness: The pregnancy rate with condom use is 0.5-7/ 100 couple-years of use. Combining condom use with spermicides is unnecessary and not cost-effective.

How to Use the Condom: Condoms should be put on before any genital contact. Air should be expelled from the tip of the condom when it is put on. The condom should be firmly held against the base of the penis during withdrawal. Condoms should not be tested before use as this may induce damage. Checking for tears before disposal is advisable.

OTHER METHODS FOR THE MALE

Other than vasectomy, the male has few choices. Under investigation are several approaches: (1) depot, nasal, or subcutaneous administration of GnRH and its analogues to suppress spermatogenesis indirectly; (2) combination of testosterone and other preparations to suppress gonadotropins; and (3) agents such as gossypol that directly interfere either with sperm motility or fertilizing capacity. These are years away from release to the market.

VASECTOMY

Vasectomy should be considered a permanent procedure. It is safe, simple, and effective (less than 2 vasectomies in 100 fail), takes less than 15 minutes and only requires local anesthesia. The incision of the vas deferens is done through a small incision made in the scrotum. At least 15 ejaculations are needed to clear sperm from the reproductive tract, so another contraceptive method should be used for at least 6 weeks.

Side-Effects: Swelling, bruising, and pain are present in 50% of men undergoing vasectomy and disappear in about 2 weeks. Other side effects are rare (less than 1%): hematoma, epididymitis, hydrocele, vasocutaneous fistula, and infection. Vasectomized men usually report either no change or an improvement in sexual behavior.

Reversal: About 2 in 1000 vasectomized men request reversal. Patency is restored in 67-100%. However, pregnancy rates after reversal range 16-85%. A large proportion of vasectomized men develop antibodies to sperm, which may reduce fertility after reversal, even with a normal count.

FOR THE FEMALE

HORMONAL CONTRACEPTION

Combined Oral Contraceptives

The oral contraceptive (OC) is the most effective form of reversible contraception available today, with a failure rate of less than 0.5 pregnancies for 100 women years. However, only 50 to 70% of the women who start taking the pill are still using it after a year.

How Do They Act: Combined OCs inhibit ovulation and interfere with reproduction at various levels:

1) Hypothalamus/pituitary level - suppression of the midcycle pituitary LH surge (basal concentration of LH and urinary excretion are not altered); FSH levels are more readily suppressed than LH levels, but the combined OC suppresses both hormones.
2) Ovary - follicular development with ovulation is prevented.
3) Endometrium - the endometrium may be inactive or irregularly secretory, inadequate for normal implantation.
4) Cervix - mucus remains thick preventing the passage of spermatozoa.

Low dose OCs contain a decreased amount of estrogen in order to make them safer. Although for most women low dose OCs are as effective in preventing pregnancy as the standard dose pill, breakthrough bleeding (BTB) may occur with greater frequency.

Biphasic or triphasic preparations may be chosen to imitate the hormonal pattern of the menstrual cycle. Total dose per cycle will be less than in most conventional OCs. The initial dosage is low followed by a step-up increment later in the cycle which helps to prevent BTB and spotting.

HORMONE CONTENT OF TRIPHASIC AND BIPHASIC OCs

Cycle Days

Triphasic	1 to 6	7 to 11	12 to 21
L Norgestrel (mg)	.050	.075	.125
Ethinyl Estradiol (µg)	30	40	30

Biphasic	1 to 10	11 to 21
Norethindrone (mg)	.05	1.0
Ethinyl Estradiol (µg)	35	35

Contraindications

1. Thromboembolic disorder or history
2. Cerebrovascular accident or history
3. Coronary artery disease or history
4. Known or suspected estrogen dependent neoplasia
5. Known pregnancy
6. Liver tumor
7. Impaired liver function

Relative Contraindications

1. Hypertension
2. Diabetes
3. Severe headache or migraine
4. Active gall bladder disease
5. Cholestasis during pregnancy or Gilbert disease
6. Mononucleosis (active phase)
7. Sickle cell disease
8. Undiagnosed vaginal bleeding

9. Elective surgery within 4 weeks
10. Long-term leg cast
11. 45 years of age or older
12. 40 years old and 2nd risk factor for cardiovascular disease
13. 30 years old, smoker of 15 cigarettes a day
14. Impaired liver function within past year

Other Possible Contraindications

1. Weight gain (ten pounds or more while taking the pill)
2. Lactation
3. Patient unreliable

Observe Carefully Patients with a History of

1. Depression
2. Chloasma
3. Hair loss during pregnancy
4. Asthma
5. Epilepsy
6. Fibroid
7. Acne
8. Varicose Veins
9. Hepatitis

How to Take the Pill: In the first cycle, the pill should be started on the first day of the cycle, followed by one pill a day for 21 days. When the pill is started on the 5th day of the first cycle, a second contraceptive method should be used for the first 15 days. In subsequent cycles, the pill is taken continuously for 3 weeks, off for 1 week, on for 3 weeks, and so on.

SIDE-EFFECTS

Of Estrogens

Thromboembolic complications
Chloasma
Nausea
Benign hepatoma
Fluid retention
Alteration in glucose tolerance tests
Decreased LDL and increased HDL cholesterol
Increased incidence of gall bladder disease

Of Progestins

Hypertension
Acne, oily skin
Depression
Cholestatic jaundice
Headache between pill cycles or when on the placebo
Decreased HDL and increased triglycerides

Thromboembolic complications (blood clots, stroke, and heart attack) are higher in women who smoke, are older than 35 years, with a history of hypertension, diabetes, heart or vascular disease. Danger signs are severe abdominal pain, severe chest pain, severe leg pain, severe headache, and blurred vision.

Choosing the Pill: A standard dose pill may be chosen if patient or physician have concerns about spotting or failure to have withdrawal bleeding with low dose OC, acne, BTB with low dose, symptoms of menopause or low estrogen levels, and when Phenytoin or Rifampin are being taken together with the pill.

Choosing between low-dose pills: When androgenic effects like hirsutism or acne are present, a less androgenic pill should be used. Demulen is one of the least androgenic pills.

Androgenic potency of progestins: Norethinodrel (0.0) < Ethinodiol Diacetate (1.01) < Norethindrone (1.60) < Norethindrone Acetate (2.50) < Norgestrel (7.60). When androgenic effects may be useful (spotting present), the most androgenic pill will be Nordette or Lo Ovral.

Estrogenic Potency of Progestins: Norgestrel (0.0) < Norethindrone (.25) < Norethindrone Acetate (.38) < Ethynodiol Diacetate (.86) < Norethynodrel (2.08).

Common Complaints and How to Deal With Them: Spotting (if related to the pill), will not last more than 3 months. The pill should be taken at a fixed time each day. For late spotting, switch to a higher progestin pill; for early spotting, raise estrogenic potency of progestin.

Failure to bleed, switch to higher progestin pill, (Ovral, Nordette, Norlestrin, Demulen); if necessary, try a higher estrogen-containing pill such as Norinyl, 1/80, Ortho Novum 1/80.
　　Hypertension, switch to a progestin only pill ("minipill").
　　Nausea, switch to a pill with less estrogen content or a "minipill."
　　Cyclic weight gain due to fluid retention, switch to a pill with less estrogen content.
　　Acne, oily skin, chronic weight gain due to increased appetite, switch to a less androgenic pill.
　　Depression, answer the obvious question, "is the depression due to the pill"
　　Headache, a detailed history is first needed. If a vascular etiology is suspected, the pill should be stopped.

NONCONTRACEPTIVE BENEFITS OF THE PILL

Protection against pelvic inflammatory disease (PID)
Improves benign breast disease
After 12 months, protection against ovarian carcinoma and
  endometrial carcinoma
Decreased cyclic problems like cramps, blood loss,
  mittelschmerz
Protection against ectopic pregnancy
Protection against ovarian cysts
Protection against anemia

Continuous Progestogen Only Pills ("Minipill")

Pregnancies are prevented by changes in the cervical mucus and
the endometrium. Forty percent of women have ovulatory cycles
during minipill use and 20% shift back and forth to and from
ovulation.

Effectiveness: Pregnancy rates with the minipill are 1.1-3.2/
100 women years. Pregnancy rates are higher in the first 6 months.

When to Prescribe a Progestin Only Pill: The minipill is
reserved for women who present estrogen-related side-effects with
the combined OC, are hypertensive, are breast feeding (fewer effects
on lactation), are over 40 years of age, present with migraine
headaches or significant history, have varicose veins.

How to Take the Minipill: Pills should be taken every day,
starting less than 4-6 weeks postpartum.

Side effects of progestin-only pills include: Irregular
menses, less menstrual flow and/or spotting, amenorrhea.

When pregnancy occurs while the patient is on the minipill, the
possibility of an ectopic pregnancy must be considered.

Postcoital Interception (PCI)

PCI is the prevention of implantation postfertilization
accomplished through luteolysis and inadequate endometrial
development.

Regimens include EE, Premarin, estrone or DES given bid in large doses, or two Ovral pills taken on two occasions 12 hours apart within 72 hours of unprotected coitus. PCI may also be accomplished with IUD insertion within 5 days of unprotected intercourse.

It is important to remember when counseling that unplanned pregnancies are not always unwanted pregnancies.

Effectiveness: The chances of becoming pregnant in cases of unprotected sexual intercourse are between 2-4% and 15-30%. Pregnancy rates are 0.7% for estrogens only regimens and 1.6% for the Ovral approach. However, the amount of EE consumed with the Ovral regimen is 125-fold less when compared with an EE regimen, with less number of tablets consumed.

Side-Effects: Nausea and vomiting occur in 53% of women with any regimen. Menorrhagia (10%) and mastalgia (20%) with estrogen only regimens are less than 1% with the Ovral regimen.

IUD

IUDs are plastic devices that can be stretched into a straight rod for insertion through the cervical canal (dilatation is not necessary). Once released into the uterine cavity the IUD resumes its original loop, spiral or T or 7 shape.

Possible mechanism of action for IUDs include: lysis or immobilization of sperm; lysis or disruption of blastocyst; eliciting an inflammatory response; prevention or disruption of implantation by inducing an increased synthesis of prostaglandins; increasing the rate of movement of the ovum in the Fallopian tube; competition with estrogens at the endometrium level by copper containing IUDs; and/or inhibition of enzyme action.

Effectiveness: Pregnancy rates are 2-4/100 women years. The physician's acceptance of the method has a strong influence on patient's acceptance and removal rate.

IUD models are: Lippes loop in 4 sizes (A, B, C, and D); the larger versions have lower rates of pregnancy and expulsion, but more removals for pain and bleeding than smaller ones (A or B). The efficacy of the smaller IUDs is improved by the addition of copper or progesterone to the new devices: Saf T Coil, Copper T, Copper 7, Nova T and Progestasert. The only IUD available in the United States is the Progestasert.

Progestasert is a T-shaped IUD which releases progesterone contained in the vertical stem of the T. Pregnancy rates are 1.8/100 women years for parous women, and removal rate, due to BTB and pain, 12.3/100 women years. Although pain and BTB may occur, a lessening of menstrual flow following insertion of Progestasert has been reported. The negative effect of progesterone and prostaglandin synthesis may result in alleviation of dysmenorrhea.

Contraindications: Pregnancy and active infection. Multiple sexual partners and frequent infections are strong relative contraindications as well as a history of ectopics, abnormal bleeding, impaired response to infection and impaired coagulation. Concern for future fertility, fibroids, valvular heart disease, cervical stenosis, small uterus, severe dysmenorrhea, severe menorrhagia, anemia, polyps, bicornuate uterus, and a history of fainting are other factors to be considered.

Side-Effects and Complications: Fifteen percent of women will have their IUD removed for spotting, bleeding, hemorrhage or anemia, and 5-20% will expel their IUD spontaneously.

With cramping and pain; infection and ectopic pregnancy should be ruled out. Pain related to the IUD may be treated with prostaglandin inhibitors or aspirin. A smaller IUD may be the answer.

If the string cannot be seen or felt, ultrasound will identify the IUD location and exclude pregnancy. If the IUD is inside the uterus it can be left in place or removed with alligator forceps, hooks, or hysteroscopy.

One-third of pregnancies with the IUD are due to undetected expulsion. If the string is visible, the IUD should be removed, which is associated with a two-fold increased risk of spontaneous abortion. When the string is not visible, ultrasound will localize the IUD or determine if unnoticed expulsion occurred. If the IUD is present, the patient should be informed of the risk of septic abortion and death should the pregnancy continue.

Women who have IUDs are less likely to experience an ectopic pregnancy than nonusers of contraception, but should pregnancy occur in an IUD wearer, it will be ectopic in about 5% of the cases.

The risk of hospitalization for women using the IUD is 1.6 as compared with women not using contraception. The presence of actinomyces (anaerobe, Gram-positive) in the uterus is associated with the use of the IUD. Unilateral ovarian abscess have been reported in IUD users.

For and Against the IUD

    PRO: high level of effectiveness
               only a single visit to a health care office required for
                    long-term use
               reversible
               no need for daily intake as the pill or consistent use as
                    barrier methods
               high rate of continuous use (a clinic visit would be
                    required to discontinue the use)
               does not have known systemic metabolic effects (can be
                    used irrespective of age, smoking, or hypertension)

    CON: increased menstrual blood loss
               pain and dysmenorrhea
               perforation
               complications of pregnancy
               increased risk of upper genital tract infection of PID
                    which can cause permanent sterility and increase the
                    risk of subsequent ectopic pregnancy (on the other
                    hand, barrier methods and OCs offer protection
                    against PID)

The IUD can be considered a useful and effective method of contraception for parous women having completed their family, who do not want to undergo sterilization, women who are over the age of 35 years are exposed to higher risk if they smoke and take OCs and the effectiveness of the IUD will be increased.

FEMALE STERILIZATION

Female sterilization should be considered an irreversible procedure only advisable for women who have completed their family or present health problems or eugenic considerations. Laparoscopy or minilaparotomy can both be used for electrical coagulation, application of a small Silastic rubber band (Falope Ring) or application of a plastic and metal clip (Hulka clip).

Minilaparotomy can be used to remove a loop of tube after ligation.

Effectiveness: Pregnancy may occur once in 400 tubal ligations and is less likely after electrocoagulation. About half of such pregnancies are ectopic.

Reversal: Reanastomosis of the tubes requires a long and expensive microsurgical procedure. Subsequent intratubal pregnancies can be expected in about 60% of cases.

Other Procedures: Hysterectomy, when there is another indication for removal of the uterus. Silastic rubber injected into the tubes using a hysteroscope and removable without surgery is being studied.

PREGNANCY TERMINATION

Contraception is preventive medicine and abortion is an answer to failure of contraceptive methods or failure to use contraception. Family planning counselling is not available in some underdeveloped countries and even in developed ones, minors are frequently unable to obtain contraception services. On the other hand, abortion is available in all societies, whether legal and safe, or illegal and dangerous, or illegal and expensive.

The risk of death from legal abortion in the United States is much less than the risk of death from continued pregnancy. Primary cause of abortion related deaths are infection (26%), embolus (26%), anesthesia (15%), hemorrhage (9.6%), coagulopathy (6.7%), preexisting cardiac disease (3.9%), electrolyte imbalance (1.9%), cerebrovascular accident (1.9%), and others (7.7%).

Complications of abortion procedures are retained tissue, infection, perforation, hematometra, continued pregnancy, cervical trauma, agglutination of the cervical canal and hemorrhage. Preabortal screening, examination of the products of conception and a careful technique including routine curettage under local anesthesia after fetal abortion will reduce later complications.

Reported long-term complications of abortion are infertility, premature delivery, and low birth weight infants.

Pregnancy termination with a progesterone antagonist (RU486) alone or combined with prostaglandins is being studied in several clinical trials with an effectiveness of about 85% for early pregnancy.

VAGINAL CONTRACEPTION

Vaginal methods, which include foams, jellys, and creams have no serious systemic side-effects. They provide some protection against STD and some of them require no prescription. However, they may be awkward to use and are less effective than oral contraceptives.

Spermicides

Spermicides (nonoxynol-9, octoxynol-9, menfegol) act as surfactants inactivating sperm by destroying the cell membrane. Spermicides should be used only to complement other methods since first year failure rates range 11-31%. If used alone, application of spermicide high in the vagina to cover the cervix should be repeated at every coitus. The several forms of spermicide bases have different melting times; vaginal foams and jellys require no melting time. Users should not douche for at least 6 hours after coitus. No evidence of systemic effects or congenital abnormalities have been reported with the use of spermicides.

Diaphragms

Diaphragms are shallow rubber domes with a firm flexible rim designed to block the upper vagina and entrance to the cervix. Diaphragms are used with a spermicidal jelly or cream since they may not fit well in all coital positions.

There are three major types of diaphragms: the flat spring diaphragm and the coil spring diaphragm fold flat and can be used with a plastic inserter. The arcing diaphragm folds into an arc and is easier to insert. Diaphragm sizes range 50-105 mm in diameter.

Effectiveness: First year failure rates are 2-3/100 users.

How to Use a Diaphragm: Diaphragm and spermicide (1 or 2 teaspoons placed within the dome and spread around the rim) are to be used at every coitus. Diaphragms must be left in place for at least 6 hours, but not longer than 24 hours after coitus. Proper application and fit should be checked in a follow-up visit.

Diaphragms should be cleaned and dried after use, and stored in a cold dark place. Women should be refitted annually or after pregnancy or if they gain or lose 10 pounds.

Side-Effects: Irritation caused by latex rubber and by spermicide and increased frequency of urinary tract irritation or infection have been reported. Vaginal lesions may result from use of too large a diaphragm or when the diaphragm is left in place for too long (over 24 hours).

Acceptability: Users complain about the need to handle genitals during insertion and removal, about the messiness of spermicide and the need to leave in diaphragm in place after use. The main complaint is impairment in the spontaneity of sexual relations.

Cervical Caps

A cervical cap is a device that fits over the cervix. It is especially recommended for women who cannot be fitted for a diaphragm.

There are three types of cap, the Prentif cavity rim, the Vault cap, and the Vimule cap, which have different shapes. When correctly fitted, none of these caps should touch the cervical os.

Effectiveness: Failure rates range 8-20/100 user years. The main reason for method failure is thought to be dislodgment due to poor fit or coital positions, and changes in the cervical shape.

How to Use the Cap: Caps with spermicide should be left in place at every coitus, and not removed for the next 6 hours. However, a cap can be left in place for longer than 24 hours (up to 3-5 days).

Side-Effects: Vaginal injury may occur with the Vimule cap in about 10% of the users.

Contraceptive Sponge

The polyurethane sponge contains about 1 g of nonoxynol-9. The sponge acts both to block the cervix and absorb ejaculate and also releases spermicide.

Effectiveness: Twelve months pregnancy rates range 9-27/100 women.

How to Use the Sponge: The sponge should be moistened with water and squeezed gently before insertion. It is used for a maximum of 24 hours, regardless of the frequency of intercourse, and then discarded.

Side-Effects: Only allergic-type reactions and vaginal irritation have been reported resulting in a discontinuation rate of 4% after 1 year of use.

LACTATION

The WHO defines 5 weeks as the earliest time when a fully lactating woman may conceive. Conception in the nonlactator has been seen as early as 21 days postpartum.

PREMENOPAUSE

Luteal phase length remains stable but there may be 10% of monophasic cycles at gynecologic age 35, and 34% by gynecologic age 40 to 45.

NATURAL FAMILY PLANNING

NFP is a way to plan for achieving or avoiding pregnancy by the timing or avoidance of intercourse by a couple during the fertile phase of the cycle.

Estrogens induce both the LH surge that will lead to ovulation and cervical mucus production. Since spermatozoa may survive up to 5 days in an appropriate milieu, the presence of estrogenic mucus will be the "danger sign" to alert that pregnancy may occur.

Billings Method: Women are taught to observe the mucus pattern at the vulva, relying on the sensation of wetness and lubrication. Couples must abstain for 72 hours following the day of peak mucus production.

Calendar Method: The Calendar Method fixes the first day of abstinence by substracting 18 from the shortest of the last 12 cycles, and the last day of abstinence by substracting 11 days from the longest of the last 12 cycles.

Calendar Thermal Method: This method combines the previous one with the temperature shift in the basal temperature chart. However, the thermal shift can occur as early as 2 days before or as late as 3 days after the LH peak.

274

SUGGESTED READING

Beck LR, Pope VZ: Controlled-release delivery systems for hormones. A review of their properties and current therapeutic use. Drugs 27:528, 1984.

Bracken MB: Spermicidal contraceptives and poor reproductive outcomes: The epidemiologic evidence against an association. Am J Obstet Gynecol 151:552, 1985.

Dorflinger LJ: Relative potency of progestins used in oral contraceptives. Contraception 31:557, 1985.

Grimes DA: Reversible contraception for the 1980s. JAMA 255:69, 1986.

Johnson JH: Contraception: The morning after. Fam Plann Perspect 16:266, 1984.

Liskin L: IUDs: An appropriate contraceptive for many women. Population Reports, Series B, No. 4, July, 1982.

Ory HW: Mortality associated with fertility and fertility control: 1983. Fam Plann Perspect 15:57, 1983.

Ory HW: The noncontraceptive health benefits from oral contraceptive use. Fam Plann Perspect 14:182, 1982.

North BB, Vorhauer BW: Use of the Today contraceptive sponge in the United States. Int J Fertil 30:81, 1985.

Vervest HAM, Haspels AA: Preliminary results with the antiprogestational compound RU-486 (mifepristone) for interruption of early pregnancy. Fertil Steril 44:627, 1985.

Zatuchni GI, Osborn CK: Gossypol: A possible male antifertility agent report of a workshop. Research Frontiers in Fertility Regulation, PARFR, Vol. 1, No. 4, 1981.

Chapter 23

Basics of Assays

Kevin G. Osteen, Ph.D.

INTRODUCTION

Within the specialty of gynecologic endocrinology and
infertility, the reproductive endocrine laboratory is of critical
importance in assisting the physician in patient management. The
purpose of this chapter is to detail the basics of hormone and
hormone receptor assay methodology currently in use in the modern
clinical reproductive endocrine laboratory. It is important to note
that good rapport between the laboratory and the clinician is
necessary for optimum patient care.

Most endocrine testing involves hormone measurement, so the
methodology for hormone measurement needs to be emphasized. Since
all hormones recognized to date require a specific receptor protein
to exert biologic activity, the basic methodology of hormone
receptor measurement and analysis will also be included.

THE LABORATORY AND THE PHYSICIAN

A variety of techniques have historically been used for steroid
hormone analysis. Older methods were generally colorimetric or
fluorometric, requiring an initial extraction of the hormone with an
organic solvent; these methods lack good specificity or sensitivity
and are labor intensive. Protein hormones were usually measured by
bioassay. Bioassays can be quite sensitive and specific, however,
they are also far too labor intensive for general use. The
introduction of radioimmunoassay (RIA) by Yalow and Berson (1960)
revolutionized the field of endocrinology as a discipline and the
role of the clinical laboratory in the diagnosis and treatment of
endocrine pathology. RIA allows for the relatively straightforward
measurement of the low circulating levels of hormones with a high
degree of specificity for the hormone of interest.

276

Although rapid analysis of hormone levels is now possible and generally expected by the physician, the most rapid tests are not always the most accurate or sensitive. Also, not all laboratories are in agreement as to the "best" methodology for a particular assay. The required quality control program within individual laboratories ensure the validity and reproducibility of assay results, however, different methodologies can lead to a rather broad range of "normal" values. The Laboratory Director should make available the appropriate information regarding normal ranges as well as the quality control data for a particular assay. The individual physician must then become acquainted with this information in order to interpret laboratory results correctly.

HORMONE ANALYSIS

Appropriateness of Sample

The laboratory cannot assure that a reported hormone level is clinically relevant. Many hormones are secreted with a diurnal rhythm and their levels in blood or urine vary as a function of the time of day. Other hormones are secreted in a pulsatile fashion resulting in significant changes in circulating levels over rather short time periods. Still other hormone levels vary with the nutritional, endocrine, or general health status of a patient. The Laboratory Director may be consulted as to appropriate sampling times, but the requesting physician must be aware of these sources of hormonal variation.

The particular laboratory test to be run determines sample collection, preparation, transport and storage. Plasma may be required instead of serum. ACTH, for example, is generally measured in plasma and must be collected in a precooled tube and kept on ice for transport to the laboratory. Certain steroids, such as pregnenolone, are also frequently measured in plasma instead of serum. Gonadotropins and gonadal steroids are usually measured by RIA in serum samples. Samples of serum once separated from the clot may be kept in a refrigerator for 2-3 days before analysis. However, storage for longer periods of time requires freezing. Protein hormones (especially follicle stimulating hormone [FSH]) do not tolerate freeze-thaw very well and consequently should be assayed as soon as possible after thawing and not be refrozen. Other considerations, such as the amount of sample needed for assay, may present special requirements of which the requesting physician needs to be aware. Laboratories should supply the appropriate information within their laboratory reference manual.

Types of Hormone and Hormone Receptor Assays: Binding Assays

        Most modern assays for hormones and their receptors use some
type of binding molecule. This binding molecule may be:

                    1) an antibody (immunoassay)
                    2) a naturally occurring binding protein
                       (competitive protein binding assay)
                    3) a specific cell receptor protein (receptor
                       binding assay).

In the case of the receptor protein, the binding assay can be
modified in order to identify or quantitate the receptor protein
itself. Common binding assays in current use include:

    Radioimmunoassay (RIA) - by far the most common of the
    binding assays used for measuring hormones, these assays use
    specific antibodies directed against the hormone of interest
    as the binding agent. Either the hormone or the antibody
    may be radioactively labeled.

    Enzyme Immunoassay (EIA) - uses an enzyme linked to the
    hormone instead of a radioactive label. The enzyme can also
    be linked to the antibody or other binder (ELIZA). The
    activity of the enzyme in the bound or free fraction can be
    quantitated by conventional chemical means following the
    binding assay.

    Fluorescent Immunoassay - uses fluorescent compounds to
    label the hormone or antibody. The degree of fluorescence
    in the bound or free fraction can be quantitated in a
    spectrofluorometer following the binding assay.

    Protein-Binding Assays - uses naturally occurring serum
    binding proteins as binding agent. These proteins (such as
    serum steroid binding proteins) are not always readily
    available in sufficient quantity for widespread use, and
    often then must be purified before they can be used.

    Hormone Receptor Binding Assay - uses the naturally
    occurring cellular receptor for a hormone as the binding
    agent. These assays have the theoretical advantage of
    representing the "true physiologic" binding ability of a
    particular hormone, but suffer from the same technical
    constraints as the other assay systems which require
    material which is difficult to obtain.

278

The classic RIA is the workhorse of the diagnostic endocrine laboratory, and should be understood. The basic principle of RIA can be applied to all binding assays.

BINDING REACTIONS DURING RIA

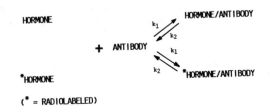

(* = RADIOLABELED)

Labeled and unlabeled hormone react in identical fashion when combined with an antibody with a high affinity and specificity for the hormone. The rate constant of the formation of the hormone-antibody complex is denoted by k_1. The reverse reaction is denoted by k_2 which represents the rate constant of the dissociation of the hormone-antibody complex.

Basic RIA Methodology

To run an RIA, the following reagents are prepared:

1) specific antibody in a known concentration
2) radiolabeled hormone, called "tracer"
3) standards (known amounts of unlabeled hormone)
4) unknowns (samples to be assayed)
5) terminating solution (precipitating reagent, etc.)

A limiting amount of specific antibody is combined in a series of tubes with increasing amounts of native (unlabeled) hormone standards in the presence of an excess (but constant amount) of hormone labeled with a radioisotope (usually tritium or iodine-125). Unknown samples are treated in identical fashion. An RIA is usually set up so that the antibody can bind only about 50% of the added labeled hormone in the total absence of unlabeled hormone. The reaction of hormone with antibody is allowed to reach (or approach) equilibrium. At equilibrium the rate of the forward reaction (formation of hormone/antibody complex) is equal to the reverse reaction (breakdown of the hormone/antibody complex). When equilibrium has been reached, some physiochemical method is used to separate the antibody-bound from unbound hormone. Typically, the antibody-bound fraction can be precipitated and thus separated from the unbound fraction by centrifugation. Following physical separation, the amount of radioactivity in either the bound or unbound fraction can then be determined. Since the amount of labeled hormone was kept constant, and the amount of antibody was limiting, the radioactivity associated with the antibody-bound fraction (i.e., the bound labeled hormone) is decreased in a relative fashion by inclusion of increasing amounts of unlabeled hormone in the assay. The amount of radioactivity in the unbound fraction has an inverse relationship to that in the antibody-bound fraction.

A standard curve can be constructed which relates the radioactivity level of individual assay tubes to the amount of native hormone that was present.

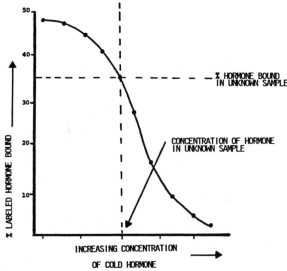

Unknown samples that were prepared in similar fashion to the native hormone "standards" are compared with these standards as to their ability to displace the labeled hormone. The amount of hormone in an unknown sample can be "read" along the standard curve by extrapolating the radioactivity associated with the particular unknown to that of a comparable standard. The principle of an RIA, thus, can be expressed in general terms as follows:

A constant amount of antibody (binder) with a sufficiently high affinity for a hormone will at equilibrium exhibit a ratio of

bound to free hormone which is quantitatively related to the
total amount of hormone in the assay tube.

Limitations of Binding Assays

Immunoassays and other binding assays now provide for the
rapid, accurate measurement of very low levels of circulating
hormones. There are, nevertheless, some limitations of this
methodology:

1. The standards used for an assay may not be identical to
   native hormone.
2. Many protein standards are not available in chemically pure
   form and must be calibrated against some form of reference
   preparation. If more than one reference preparation is in
   current use, the particular reference preparation used must
   be stated in order to interpret a laboratory value. An
   important example of this situation exists for human
   chorionic gonadotropin (hCG). Two calibration standards
   are in current use for hCG RIA. These reference
   preparations, the 2nd IS (Second International Standard)
   and the 1st IRP (First International Reference Preparation)
   are quite different. The 1st IRP is the most recent
   preparation, but the least frequently used. Values for
   assays calibrated against each preparation are reported
   in mIU's but differ by about two-fold depending on the
   specificity of the antibody used.
3. Metabolites or subunits of some hormones often possess
   immunoreactivity and, thus, their presence in a sample
   would falsely elevate a laboratory result from an
   immunoassay.
4. Interfering substances that bind hormones in a biologic
   sample may prevent the detection of a certain amount of
   hormone and falsely lower a laboratory result. Serum
   steroid-binding proteins are an example.
5. Antibodies, binding proteins, and receptors do not have
   absolute specificity for their respective hormone and,
   thus, cross-reactivity of these binders with related
   hormones falsely elevates a result.
6. Patients who have undergone radiotherapy may have residual
   radioactivity in their system which would interfere with
   any binding assay based on a radiolabeled constituent.

HORMONE RECEPTOR ASSAYS

Receptors can be used as binder in receptor binding assays for
both steroid and protein hormones. Uterine cytosol preparations can

be used in receptor binding assays for estradiol, and rat testis can be used to measure LH/hCG. Binding assays using native hormone receptors are not routinely used for hormone analysis in the clinical laboratory for technical reasons. However, receptor binding is used extensively in both the research and clinical setting to identify and characterize hormone receptors in target tissues. Receptor number and the receptor's affinity for its respective hormone (the K value) can be calculated from the data obtained from a "standard curve" which has been redrawn according to the Scatchard Plot.

The interaction between a hormone (H) and its receptor (R) is similar to the hormone-antibody reaction.

$$H + R \rightleftarrows HR$$

The Law of Mass Action dictates that at equilibrium the concentrations of the products on each side of the above kinetic equation will be a constant ratio. This constant (K) then becomes:

$$\frac{[HR]}{[H][R]} = K$$

In this equation [HR], [H] and [R] represent the concentrations of the bound (numerator) and free (denominator) components at equilibrium. Since the concentrations of H and R at equilibrium are really the total concentrations of these components minus that part in the bound fraction, we can express K as follows:

$$\frac{[HR]}{[H-HR][R-HR]} = K$$

If we substitute X for HR, multiply both sides of the equation by (R-X) and then rearrange the equation into the form of Y = MX - B (the equation for a straight line with a negative slope) we get:

$$\frac{X}{(H-X)} = K R - KX$$

Since both K and R are constant values the variable becomes a minus KX. As seen below, the plot of this equation gives a straight line with a slope of minus K.

282

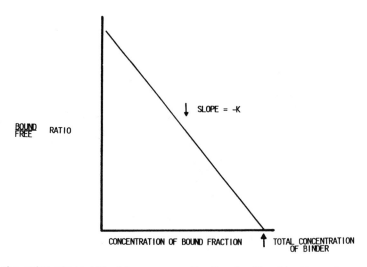

SLOPE = -K

BOUND/FREE RATIO

CONCENTRATION OF BOUND FRACTION ↑ TOTAL CONCENTRATION OF BINDER

At the point where this line crosses the Y axis (Y = 0), the value
of KR - KX = 0. This equation can be rearranged to KR = KX which
reduces to R = X. Thus, both receptor number and K can be
calculated from the Scatchard Plot. The Scatchard Plot assumes a
single class of binding sites in order to produce a straight line.
This condition is not always met in biologic systems; nevertheless,
the Scatchard analysis does provide useful information which is
often of clinical significance.

UNITS OF HORMONE MEASUREMENT

Values for hormone levels may be reported differently by
various clinical laboratories. The "units" that a particular
laboratory reports thus may be a source of some confusion if the
physician is unfamiliar with systems of measure in common use.
Three common sources of confusion and a brief clarification of each
are included here.

1) "International Units" (IU) or milli-International Units
(mIU) vs mass units such as ng/ml or μg/ml.

Many hormones are either not available in pure form or are
unavailable in sufficient quantities as pure hormone for
general use. Also in many blood samples, the hormones of
interest may be present as isoforms (for example,
gonadotropins that differ in their carbohydrate moities) or
in various states of degradation or incomplete synthesis. It

is therefore necessary that some agreement be made as to what
to call "hCG" or "LH" in a sample containing the above
mixture. This problem has been addressed by various national
and international agencies such as the Expert Committee on
Biological Standardization of the World Health Organization.
These agencies establish "reference preparations" to which
the standards to be used in an actual assay can be calibrated.
Therefore, a hormone level that is reported in IU/ml or
mIU/ml has been measured by an assay system which has been
calibrated against a reference preparation. A hormone level
that is reported in ng/ml or some other mass unit has
utilized a highly purified standard which may or may not have
been calibrated against a reference preparation. Again, the
laboratory director or the laboratory handbook should be
consulted in order to interpret results reported in either
fashion.

2) Reporting of mass units as "percent" solutions (μg% or
μmole%) vs mass per volume (pg/ml or ng/ml).

When purified hormone for standardization is available, most
laboratories report blood hormone levels in terms of mass per
unit volume such as pg/ml (picogram[s] per milliliter) or
ng/dl (nanogram[s] per deciliter). However, some
laboratories may report their results as a percent such as
ng% (nanogram percent). Though it is not entirely correct to
express a value in this fashion, it is a simple matter to
convert these values to mass per unit volume. For example,
10 ng% = 10 ng/dl or 0.1 ng/ml (the percent implies "per 100
milliliters").

3) Unfamiliarity of the physician with the common prefixes for
units of measure such as pg vs ng.

Common units of mass and volume used by clinical laboratories
are listed in the table below.

Power of 10	Volume unit	Mass unit
unit	liter (L)	gram (g)
10^{-1}	deciliter (dl)	decigram (dg)
10^{-2}	centiliter (cl)	centigram (cg)
10^{-3}	milliliter (ml)	milligram (mg)
10^{-6}	microliter (μl)	microgram (μg)
10^{-9}	nanoliter (nl)	nanogram (ng)
10^{-12}	picoliter (pl)	picogram (pg)
10^{-15}	femtoliter (fl)	femtogram (fg)

It is important to note here again that even if different
clinical laboratories report their measurements using the same
"units," normal ranges are established within each individual
laboratory. Therefore, the physician must still consult the
laboratory in order to appreciate fully the significance of a
laboratory result.

SUGGESTED READING

Chard T: An introduction to radioimmunoassay and related techniques.
In: Work TS, Work E (eds): Laboratory Techniques in Biochemistry
and Molecular Biology. New York, Elsevier Biomedical, 1986.

Rodbard D: Mathematics of hormone-receptor interation, I. Basic
principals. In: O'Malley BW, Means AR (eds): Receptors for
Reproductive Hormones, New York, Plenum, 1973, pp 289-326. (Adv Exp
Med Biol 36)

Rosenberg E: Selection of standards for the measurement of
pituitary hormones: Problems of standardization. In: Ligan J,
Clapp JJ (eds): Ligand Assay, Analysis of International
Developments on Isotopic and Non-Isotopic Immunoassay: New York,
Masson Publishing USA, Inc, 1981, pp 31-43.

INDEX

Abortion, 200, 270 (see also
    Miscarriage)
  complications of, 270
  incomplete, 38
  spontaneous, 216-217, 234
    chromosome anomalies in, 235-236
    in in vitro fertilization, 253
Abruptio placenta, 243
Acetylcholine, 45
Acrosin assay, 229
ACTH, 8, 98-100
  in adrenal insufficiency, 106
  excess, 107, 108, 109
  measurement of, 276
  secretion of, 110
  syndrome, 103
ACTH stimulation test, 73, 77, 101,
    102, 105
Addison's disease, 103-107
Adenomas, testosterone producing, 78
Adenomyosis, 63, 213
Adrenal adenoma, 11
Adrenal carcinoma, 111-112
Adrenal cortex, 6
Adrenal corticosteroids, 33
Adrenal glands (see also Cushing's
    syndrome)
  autoimmune destruction of, 103
  function of, 98-101
  insufficiency, 103-107
  mass in, 111-112
  output measurement, 100-101
  stimulation tests of, 101-102
  suppression tests of, 102-103
Adrenal hyperplasia, 12, 107, 111
    (see also CAH-ACTH stimula-
    tion test)
  congenital (CAH), 20, 33
  hirsutism and, 76-78
Adrenal steroidogenesis, 6-8
Adrenal suppression, 79, 80
Adrenal tumor, 39, 78
Adrenalectomy, 110
α-Adrenergic neurons, 5
Adrenocortical carcinoma, 111
Aging, estrogen deficiency and, 126
Alcohol, fetotoxic effects of, 238
Aldosterone, 98
  inadequate, 20
  regulation of, 8

Allergies and premenstrual
    syndrome, 120
Amenorrhea
  definition of, 28
  exercise-related, 41-42
  gonadal, 42-43
  with hyperprolactinemia, 55
  hypothalamic, 41, 159
  incidence of, 48
  ovulation induction for,
    148, 149
  pituitary, 42
  primary, 28-29
    etiology of, 29-30
    evaluation of, 31
    laboratory work-up for,
      31-33
    treatment of, 33
  secondary, 33-34
    differential diagnosis
      of, 36-43
    etiology of, 34
    evaluation of, 34-43
    laboratory studies of,
      35-36
  stress-associated, 42
Amniocentesis, 254
Anabolic steroids, 79
Anagen, 68
Anatomic abnormalities, 24
Androgen insensitivity
    syndrome, 23
Androgen producing tumors, 21
Androgenic steroids, 29
Androgens, 6
  hair growth and, 69, 70
  inadequate, 21
  measurement of, 49
  for menorrhagia, 63
  premenstrual syndrome and,
    119
  ring structure of, 9
  synthesis defects of, 23
Androstane, 6
3-Androstanediol-glucuronide,
    73
Androstenedione
  circulating, 71
  conversion of, 70
  decrease of in menopause,
    126

290

Epididymis, 15, 162
Epididymitis, 230
Estradiol, 1-2, 8, 136
  decreasing, 125
  effects of, 3
  in luteal phase, 4
  measuring, 230
  for menopause, 134
  metabolism of, 10
  in ovulation, 4
  in premenstrual syndrome, 120
  progesterone and, 197
Estratriene, 6
Estriols, 134
  biologic potency of, 135
Estrogen (see also Estrogen
      replacement therapy)
  biologic potency of, 135-136
  with clomiphene citrate
      therapy, 151
  conjugated, 137
  deficiency, 126
  inadequate milieu, 196,223
  for intrauterine adhesions, 193
  metabolic pathways of, 11
  metabolism if, 133
  pathways of, 10
  premenstrual syndrome and, 129
  protective effect of, 138
  release of, 29
  side effects of, 264
  stimulation of, 33
  synthetic, 135
  thyroid-binding globulin and,
      95-96
  types of, 134
Estrogen analogues, synthetic, 134
Estrogen receptor synthesis, 196
Estrogen replacement therapy
  for amenorrhea, 43
  benefits of, 129-132
  contraindications to, 132-133
  for endometriosis, 213, 214, 222,
      224
  indications for, 129
  risk:benefit ration with, 132
  risks and complications of,
      133-134
  for spontaneous miscarriage,
      240
Estrogenic mucus, 273

Estrogen-progesterone provo-
      cative test, 38
Estrone, 134
  biologic potency of, 135
  in contraception, 267
  conversion to, 136
  in menopause, 126
  metabolism of, 10
Estrone sulfate, 135
Ethynodiol diacetate, 265
Ethinyl estradiol, 33, 135
Ethisterone, 21
Exercise
  amenorrhea and, 41-42
  bone loss from, 43
  for menopause therapy, 137
  for premenstrual syndrome,
      120
  strenuous, 200

Family planning, 273
Fecundity, 140
  in amenorrhea, 33
Female differentiation, 14-15
Female external genitalia
  abnormal formation of, 20
  differentiation of, 15, 16
Female infertility, 230-231
  (see also Infertility)
Female pseudohermaphroditism,
      19
Fertility (see Fecundity;
      Infertility)
Fibrinolysis, 205
Fibroids, 193-194
  submucous, 237
Fimbrial agglutination, 208
Fimbrioplasty, 208
Flat capillary tube penetra-
      tion tests, 186-187
Fluid and electrolyte therapy,
      105
Fluid volume, extracellular, 8
Fluorescent immunoassay, 277
Fluorescent techniques, 32
Fluoride, 137
Foley catheter, 193, 194, 240
Follicle
  antral, 2-3
  degeneration of, 15
  development monitoring of,
      249-250

therapy for, 241
trimester, 194
Pregnane, 6
Pregnanediol, 11
Pregnanetriol, 12
Pregnenolone, 8, 21, 276
Premarin, 33, 38, 62, 267
Premature delivery, 193, 236
Premenstrual staining, 63
Premenstrual syndrome, 117
  diagnosis of, 120
  etiology of, 118-120
  incidence of 118
  treatment for, 120-123
Premenstrual tension, 117
Preovulatory follicle, 3
Primitive zygotes, 13-14
Primordial follicle, 2
Progestational agent
  for abnormal bleeding, 60
  in amenorrhea treatment, 40
  bleeding and, 62
  for congenital uterine anomalies, 194
  for premenstrual staining, 63
Progesterone
  for abnormal bleeding, 59, 60
  allergic reaction to, 120
  bioassay of output, 199-200
  decrease in, 113
  high, 32-33
  inadequacy of, 196
  increase in, 3
  in luteal phase, 4
  masculinization effect of, 21
  measurement of, 196-197, 230
  metabolic pathways of, 11
  negative effects of, 268
  in ovulation, 4
  for premenstrual staining, 63
  premenstrual syndrome and, 118, 121
  secretion of, 1, 8
  spontaneous miscarriage and, 236
  stimulation of bleeding with, 37-38
  substitution therapy, 201, 203
  suppositories, 62, 159, 195, 203
  uterine congenital anomalies and, 193, 203
  withdrawal from, 148

Progesterone receptor defect, 196
Progesterone supplementation
  for luteal phase inadequacy, 241-242
Progesterone test for amenorrhea, 37
Progestin
  for endometriosis, 222, 223, 224
  side effects of, 264, 265
  hirsutism and, 79, 81
  masculinization effect of, 21
  in menopause therapy, 136-138
  for premenstrual syndrome, 121
Progestogen in contraceptives, 266
Prolactin
  elevated, 47, 49, 172
  inhibitory control of, 45, 95
  for premenstrual syndrome, 120
  restoration of, 156
  serum level, 36
  stimulation of, 2
  suppression of, 50, 157
Prolactin inhibiting factor (PIF), 45
Prolactinomas
  problems of, 55
  treatment of, 52
Prolactin-producing pituitary tumor, 36
Promethazine, 207
Propranolol, 89, 91
Propylthiouracil (PTU), 88, 89, 96
Prostaglandin
  in endometriosis, 216
  increased synthesis of, 267
  in luteal phase, 4
  menstrual fluid, 114
  negative effects of, 268
  in ovulation, 4
  premenstrual syndrome and, 120
  release of, 113

Spermatogenesis, 161-162
Sperm (see also Semen)
  abnormalities of, 241
  absence of, 172
  clumping of, 230
  decreased DNA content of, 239
  motility of, 171-172, 173, 184,
    230
  mucus penetration of, 171
Sperm agglutination testing, 189
Sperm agglutination/aggregation,
  167
Sperm count, 166, 168
  low, 172
  reduced, 174
Sperm immobilization testing, 189
Sperm maturation, 163
Sperm penetration assay, 168-169,
  176, 230
Sperm performance tests, 187, 230
Sperm rise, 179
Sperm wash, 179, 190
Spermatogenesis
  abnormalities in, 172
  defective, 167
Spermatozoa, percentage of, 171
Sperm-cervical mucus cross-match
    test, 186, 187, 189
Sperm-cervical mucus interaction,
    182, 183, 186-190
Sperm-cervical mucus penetration
    tests, 187
Spermicides, 271
Sperm-mucus incompatibility, 187
Spermocytotoxicity testing, 189
Spironolactone
  in amenorrhea treatment, 40
  for hirsutism 79, 80
  for premenstrual syndrome, 122
Split ejaculate, 179
Sterility, 140
Sterilization, female, 269-270
  reversal of, 209, 270
Steroid
  anabolic, 138
  basic ring structure of, 5-6
  biosynthetic pathways of, 7
  gonadal, 5
  high-dose, 190
  measurement of, 276
  metabolism of, 9-12

replacement, 105, 107
Steroidogenesis, 5-8
  gonadal, 8
Strassman unification, 240
Stress
  amenorrhea and, 42
  and early pregnancy wastage,
    243
  premenstrual syndrome and,
    119
Suction biopsy, 60
Sugars, refined, and
    premenstrual syndrome,
    120-121
Surgery (see also specific
    techniques)
  for Cushing's syndrome,
    109-110
  for dysmenorrhea, 116-117
  for endometriosis, 224
  factors predictive of
    success of, 55
  for hyperprolactinemia, 52
  for hyperthyroidism, 89
  microsurgical techniques in,
    206
Swyer syndrome, 19
Systemic lupus erythematosus,
    237

T_3 (see Triiodothyrione)
T_4 (see Thyroxine)
Tapazole, 88
TEBG, 74-75
Telogen, 68
Terminal hair, 68, 73
Testicular feminization, 23,
    31
Testicular regression
    syndrome, 19
Testis
  function abnormalities of,
    172
  injury to or infection of,
    163, 230
Testosterone, 8
  decrease of in menopause,
    126
  hair growth and, 70
  inadequate, 21
  increased, 34

302

levels of in tumor, 78
obesity and, 75
for premenstrual syndrome, 120
production of, 15, 16, 161
Testosterone-estradiol binding
globulin (TEBG), 70-71
TEST-yolk buffer, 169, 179
Tetrahydrometabolites, 21
Thelarche, 28, 29
Thionamides, 88, 89
Thromboembolic phenomena, 133
Thyroid stimulating hormone (TSH),
85-86
Thyrotropin-releasing hormone
(TRH), 45
Thyroidal 24-hour radioactive
iodine uptake (RAIU),
86-87
Thyroglobulin, 92
Thyroid
carcinoma, 94
changes in during pregnancy,
95-96
disorders of, 87-96 (see also
specific conditions)
function of, 83-87
imaging of, 87
in neonate, 96
nodules, 94-95
Thyroid binding globulin (TBG), 84
Thyroid dysfunction, 33
Thyroid function, 87
Thyroid releasing hormone (TRH),
86
Thyroid replacement, 93
Thyroid stimulating hormone, 49, 96
Thyroid storm, 90-91
Thyroid suppressive therapy, 95
Thyroid-binding globulin, 95-96
Thyroidectomy, 89
Thyroiditis, chronic autoimmune, 93
Thyrotropin (see Thyroid stimulating
hormone)
Thyrotropin releasing hormone (TRH),
83
Thyroxine, 83-84
elevated levels of, 87
in hypothyroidism, 91, 92, 93
maternal, 96
during pregnancy, 95-96
in thyroid storm treatment, 91

Thyroxine index, free (FTI),
85
Tompkins procedure, 240
TORCH studies, 240
Transsphenoidal pituitary
surgery, 52, 55, 109
Transvaginal USG aspiration,
250
Transverse vaginal septum, 31
TRH (see Thyrotropin-releasing
hormone)
Trichomonas, 184
Triglycerides
in hypothyroidism, 92
in menopause, 126
Triiodothyronine, 83-84
elevated levels of, 87
in hypothyroidism, 91, 92,
94
maternal, 96
resin uptake of, 84-85
in thyroid storm treatment,
91
Trophoblast/lymphocyte cross-
reactive (TLX)
antigens, 238
TSH (see Thyroid stimulating
hormone)
Tubal factor infertility,
207-211
Tubal occlusion, 209, 211
rates of, 206
Tubal patency, 210
Tubal reimplantation, 211
Tumor (see also Macroadenomas;
Microadenomas)
adrenal, 78
gonadoblastoma/dysgerminoma,
24
hirsutism and, 78
maternal androgen producing,
21
ovarian, 75, 78
pituitary, 46, 47
discovery of, 49-50
radiologic study of, 172
prolactin producing, 52
screening tests for, 78
testing for, 73
Turner's syndrome, 256
stigmata of, 17-18